Study Guide for

Nursing Research: Methods and Critical Appraisal for Evidence-Based Practice

Sixth Edition

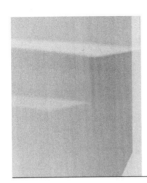

Kathleen Rose-Grippa, PhD, RN
Professor
School of Nursing
Ohio University
Athens, Ohio

Mary Jo Gorney-Moreno, PhD, RN
Associate Vice President
Academic Technology;
Professor
School of Nursing
San Jose State University
San Jose, California

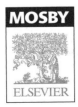

MOSBY

ELSEVIER

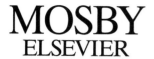

MOSBY
ELSEVIER

11830 Westline Industrial Drive
St. Louis, Missouri 63146

STUDY GUIDE
NURSING RESEARCH: METHODS AND CRITICAL APPRAISAL FOR
EVIDENCE-BASED PRACTICE, Sixth Edition

ISBN 13   9780323031707
ISBN 10   0323031706

NOTICE

Knowledge and best practice in this field are constantly changing. As new research and experience broaden our knowledge, changes in practice, treatment and drug therapy may become necessary or appropriate. Readers are advised to check the most current information provided (i) on procedures featured or (ii) by the manufacturer of each product to be administered, to verify the recommended dose or formula, the method and duration of administration, and contraindications. It is the responsibility of the practitioner, relying on their own experience and knowledge of the patient, to make diagnoses, to determine dosages and the best treatment for each individual patient, and to take all appropriate safety precautions. To the fullest extent of the law, neither the Publisher nor the Authors assumes any liability for any injury and/or damage to persons or property arising out or related to any use of the material contained in this book.

The Publisher

ISBN 13   9780323031707
ISBN 10   0323031706

Acquisitions Editor: Lee Henderson
Senior Developmental Editor: Rae L. Robertson
Book Production Manager: Gayle May

Printed in the United States of America

Last digit is the print number: 9 8 7 6 5 4 3 2 1

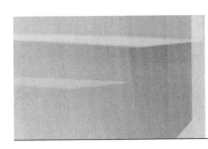

Contributors

Mary Lou DeNatale, BSN, MSN, EdD
Associate Professor of Nursing
University of San Francisco
San Francisco, California

Chapter 12, *Sampling*

Sharon A. Denham, DSN, RN
Associate Professor
School of Nursing
Ohio University
Athens, Ohio

Chapter 6, *Introduction to Qualitative Research*
Chapter 7, *Qualitative Approaches to Research*
Chapter 8, *Evaluating Qualitative Research*

Mary Jo Gorney-Moreno, PhD, RN
Associate Vice President
Academic Technology
San Jose State University
San Jose, California

Chapter 9, *Introduction to Quantitative Research*
Chapter 10, *Experimental and Quasiexperimental Designs*
Chapter 11, *Nonexperimental Designs*
Chapter 13, *Legal and Ethical Issues*

Kathleen Rose-Grippa, PhD, RN
Professor
School of Nursing
Ohio University
Athens, Ohio

Chapter 14, *Data-Collection Methods*
Chapter 15, *Reliability and Validity*
Chapter 16, *Data Analysis: Descriptive and Inferential Statistics*
Chapter 17, *Analysis of Findings*
Chapter 18, *Evaluating Quantitative Research*
Chapter 19, *Developing an Evidence-Based Practice*
Chapter 20, *Tools for Applying Evidence to Practice*

Therese Snively, PhD, RN
Assistant Professor
School of Nursing
Ohio University
Athens, Ohio

Chapter 1, *The Role of Research in Nursing*
Chapter 2, *The Research Process: Integrating Evidence-Based Practice*
Chapter 3, *Developing Research Questions and Hypotheses*
Chapter 4, *Literature Review*
Chapter 5, *Theoretical Framework*

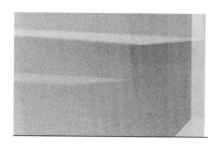

Dedication

To Paul, without whom none of it would have been possible.

To Rebekah, Carolyn, Richard, Greg, Caitlin, Lydia, Sarah, Matthew, and Michael, who have taught me to make every minute count.

To my parents, Dee and Dick, for many years of support and encouragement.

To E. Pieper, for requiring a written Christmas story with no verbs.

To all of the students who have had the courage and commitment to ask a question.

Kathy Rose-Grippa

To Kathleen Rose-Grippa, my role-model, who balances family and career with grace, wisdom, and humor.

To my husband, Manuel Moreno, thank you for your steadfast support against all odds. It is appreciated more than I can say.

Mary Jo Gorney-Moreno

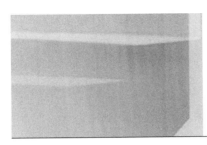

Introduction

Information bombards us! The student lament used to be "I can't find any information on X." Now the cry is "What do I do with all of the information on X?" The focus shifts from finding information to thinking about how to use information. What information is worth keeping? What should be discarded? What is useful to practice? What is fluff? Where are the gaps?

Thinking about the links between information and practice is critical to the improvement of the nursing care we deliver. As each of us strengthens our individual understanding of the links between interventions and outcomes, we move the discipline's collective practice closer to being truly evidence-based. We can "know" what intervention works best in what situation.

"Helping people get better" begins with thinking. Our intent is that the activities in the Study Guide will help you strengthen your skills in thinking about information. The activities are designed to assist you in evaluating the research you read so you are prepared to undertake the critical analysis of all research studies. As you practice the critiquing skills addressed in this Study Guide, you will be strengthening your ability to make practice-based decisions grounded in nursing theory and research.

What an incredible time to be a nurse!

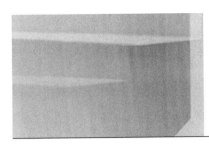

General Directions

1. Complete each chapter and the activities in that chapter sequentially. This Study Guide is designed so that you build on the knowledge gained in Chapter 1 to complete the activities in Chapter 2, and so forth. The activities are designed to give you the opportunity to apply the knowledge learned in the textbook and actually use this knowledge to solve problems, thereby gaining increased confidence that comes only from working through each chapter.

2. Follow the specific directions that precede each activity. Be certain that you have the resources needed to complete the activity before you begin that activity.

3. Do the post-test after all of the chapter's activities have been completed. The answers for the post-test items can be obtained from your instructor. If you answer 85% of the questions correctly, be confident that you have grasped the essential material presented in the chapter.

4. Clarify any questions, confusion, or concerns you may have with your instructor, or e-mail K. Rose-Grippa (grippa@ohio.edu).

5. We recommend that you read the textbook chapter first, then complete the Study Guide activities for that chapter.

Activity Answers Are in the Back of this Book

Answers in a workbook such as this are not "cut and dried" like answers in a math book. Many times you are asked to make a judgment call about a particular problem. If your judgment differs from that of the authors, review the criteria that you used to make your decision. Determine if you followed a logical progression of steps to reach your conclusion. If not, rework the activity. If the process you followed appears logical, and your answer remains different, remember that even experts may disagree on many of the judgment calls in nursing research.

There will continue to be many "gray areas." If you average an 85% agreement with the authors, you can be sure that you are on the right track and should feel very confident about your level of expertise.

Kathleen Rose-Grippa, PhD, RN
E-mail: grippa@ohio.edu

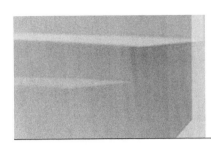

Contents

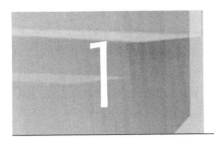

The Role of Research in Nursing

INTRODUCTION

One goal of this chapter in the study guide is to assist you in reviewing the material presented in chapter 1 of the text written by LoBiondo-Wood and Haber. A second and more fundamental goal is to provide you with an opportunity to begin practicing the role of a critical consumer of research. Succeeding chapters in this workbook fine-tune your ability to evaluate research studies critically.

LEARNING OUTCOMES

On completion of this chapter, the student should be able to do the following:

- State the significance of research to evidence-based nursing practice.
- Identify the role of the consumer of nursing research.
- Discuss the differences in trends in nursing research.
- Describe how research, education, and practice relate to each other.
- Evaluate the nurse's role in the research process as it relates to the nurse's level of educational preparation.
- Identify the future trends in nursing research.
- Formulate the priorities for nursing research in the twenty-first century.

Activity 1

Match the term in Column B with the appropriate phrase in Column A. Each term will be used only once. This may be a good time to review the glossary.

Column A

1. _____ Systematic inquiry into possible relationships among particular phenomena

2. _____ One who reads critically and applies research findings in nursing practice

3. _____ Examines the effects of nursing care on patient outcomes in a systematic process

4. _____ Critically evaluates a research report's content based on a set of criteria to evaluate the scientific merit for application

5. _____ Implementation of a scientifically sound research-based innovation into clinical practice

6. _____ Theoretical or pure research that generates tests and expands theories that explain phenomena

7. _____ Clinical practice based upon the collection, interpretation, and integration of expert knowledge, research-derived evidence, and patient preferences

Column B

a. Critique
b. Consumer
c. Research
d. Clinical research
e. Basic research
f. Evidence-based practice
g. Research utilization

Activity 2

Listed below are specific research activities. Using the American Nurses' Association (ANA) guidelines, indicate which group of nurses has the primary responsibility for each activity. Use the abbreviations from the key provided.

Key: A = Associate degree   C = Master's degree
         B = Baccalaureate degree   D = Doctoral degree

1. _____   Design and conduct research studies

2. _____   Identify nursing problems needing investigation

3. _____   Assist others in applying nursing's scientific knowledge

4. _____   Develop methods of scientific inquiry

5. _____   Assist in data collection activities

6. _____   Be a knowledgeable consumer of research

7. _____   Demonstrate an awareness of value of nursing research

8. _____   Collaborate with an experienced researcher in proposal development, data analysis, and interpretation

9. _____   Promote the integration of research into clinical practice

Activity 3

1. Examine the four articles that are in the appendices of the LoBiondo-Wood and Haber text. What is the educational preparation of the person(s) responsible for each study? List the degrees (i.e., RN, BSN, MS, PhD, or DNSc) of each author next to the author's name. Remember, this information is usually found in the short biographical paragraph on the first page or at the end of the article.

   a. Koniak-Griffin:

       Verzemnieks:

       Anderson:

       Brecht:

       Lesser:

       Kim:

       Turner-Pluta:

   b. Van Cleve:

      Bossert:

      Beecroft:

      Adlard:

      Alvarez:

      Savedra:

   c. Plach:

      Stevens:

      Moss:

   d. Davison:

      Goldenberg:

      Gleave:

      Degner:

2. In what way does this information regarding the educational preparation of the researcher influence your thinking about the study? Before drawing any conclusions, answer the following questions:

   a. Is the first author's education preparation at the doctoral level? (Circle the correct answer.)

Appendix A	Yes	No
Appendix B	Yes	No
Appendix C	Yes	No
Appendix D	Yes	No

     The general assumption is that the first author carries the major responsibility for the research.

b. If there are other authors, is there other evidence of his or her role in the research (such as data collector), and is this congruent with ANA's prescription for roles based on educational preparation?

Appendix A:

Appendix B:

Appendix C:

Appendix D:

c. Were any of the studies funded by external funding agencies? Write below which study and agency provided external funding, if any. This would indicate that the research proposal had been reviewed by an external source and deemed meritorious enough to receive funding to complete the study.

Appendix A:

Appendix B:

Appendix C:

Appendix D:

Activity 4

Complete the following crossword puzzle as you would any other crossword puzzle. Note that if more than one word is needed in an answer, there will be no blank spaces between the two (or more) words of the name or phrase. Refer to the text for help.

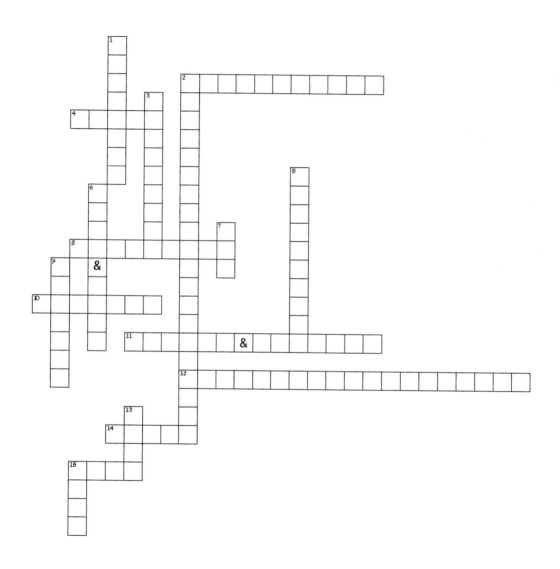

Across

2. In the 1920s, many studies using this type of research design were published in the *American Journal of Nursing* (*AJN*). (2 words)
4. Historically, this group has been excluded from clinical research and is likely to be a topic associated with major funding in the future.
8. Focus of nursing research between 1900 and 1950.
10. Researcher who conducted a classic clinically oriented study of safety and cost savings of early hospital discharge of very-low-birth-weight infants.
11. They studied aspects of thanatology, the care of dying patients, and their caretakers.
12. Collected and analyzed data on the health status of the British Army during the Crimean War.
14. Increased emphasis on practice-oriented research occurred in this decade (numerical answer).
15. Last year of the decade in which the earliest nursing research course was taught (numerical answer).

Down

1. _____ report in 1923 sponsored by the Rockefeller Foundation emphasized the need for nursing education to move into the university.
2. Focus of U.S. Public Health funded nursing research in the 1950s (abbreviate the last plural word in this answer).
3. One of the first topics of clinically oriented research in the early half of the century.
5. Lydia Hall's research led to the creation of this totally nurse-run health care facility.
6. The research of _____ and _____ led to the hiring of school nurses by New York City.
7. This organization sponsored the first Nursing Research Conference in 1967 (initials only).
9. National Center for _____ Research established in 1986 at NIH.
13. The current *Healthy People 2010* is the latest set of national health goals which began with the *Surgeon General's Report* of _____ (numerical answer).
15. First year of the decade in which the *Journal of Nursing Research* was first published (numerical answer).

Activity 5

The Department of Health and Human Services published *Healthy People 2000* in 1992. The report is a compilation of 22 expert working groups who specified as one objective: "to reduce physical abuse directed at women by male partners to no more than 27 per 1,000 couples." One example of the way nursing is helping to achieve this objective is through studies and publications such as the 1993 *Nursing Research* article, "Physical and emotional abuse in pregnancy: a comparison of adult and teenage women" by Parker. Other ways nursing and nurse researchers are helping to address this objective are:

a.

b.

c.

d.

Activity 6

Now that you have read the chapter, answer the following questions in your own words in a way that is meaningful to you.

1. Why is knowing about nursing research important?

2. How will nurses produce depth in nursing science?

3. If you were asked to give testimony about your practice to the local city council, state assembly, or senate, what research information would you like to have to assist you in presenting the testimony?

Activity 7: Web-Based Activity

Go to the website http://www.ahrq.gov/about/nursing/ and read the following:

a. About nurses at AHRQ
b. Senior Scholar in Nursing
c. Future Directions in Primary Care Research: New Special Issues for Nurses (found under Tools and Resources)

Under the title "Research Findings," choose a research activity and read the report.

Activity 8: Evidence-Based Practice Activity

A good website to learn more about evidence-based practice is the Academic Center for Evidence-Based Nursing (ACE) at the University of Texas Health Science Center at San Antonio (http://www.acestar.uthscsa.edu/). Click on "Learn about EBP" and "EBP resources." Read these sections and then identify databases that you would use in doing a literature search.

POST-TEST

1. Listed below are descriptions of research activities being carried out by nurses. Indicate in the space in front of each description for which of the following the action is most appropriate:

A = An associate degree prepared nurse
B = A baccalaureate degree prepared nurse
C = A master's prepared nurse
D = A doctorally prepared nurse

a. _____ Provide expert consulting to a unit that is considering changing the unit's practice on the care of decubitus ulcers based on the results from a series of studies.

b. _____ Take and record the blood pressures of hypertensive clients during their monthly visits to the clinic. Blood pressures are taken as part of a study on the effects of contingency contracting by a nurse researcher.

c. _____ To understand and critically appraise research studies to discriminate whether a study is provocative or whether the findings have sufficient support to be considered for utilization.

d. _____ Design and conduct research studies to expand nursing knowledge such as the Anderson (1993) study, "The Parenting Profile Assessment: Screening for Child Abuse."

2. Match the terms in Column B with the appropriate phrase in Column A. Not all terms from Column B will be used.

Column A

1. _____   First nursing doctoral program began at Teacher's College, Columbia University

2. _____   National Institute for Nursing Research authorized

3. _____   Nightingale studied mortality rates of British in Crimean War

4. _____   NINR areas of special interest for these years include testing community-based nursing models

5. _____   *Nursing Research* publication began

Column B

a. 1995 to 1999
b. Mid and late 19th century
c. 1992
d. 1920 to 1929
e. 1993
f. 1952
g. 1900
h. 2000

Please check with your instructor for the answers to the post-test.

REFERENCES

Anderson CL (1993). The parenting profile assessment: Screening for child abuse, *Appl Nurs Res* 6(1):31-38.

Davison BJ, Goldenberg SL, Gleave ME, et al. (2003). Provision of individualized information to men and their partners to facilitate treatment decision making in prostate cancer, *Oncol Nurs Forum* 30(1):107-114.

Koniak-Griffin D, Verzemnieks IL, Anderson NLR, et al. (2003). Nurse visitation for adolescent mothers: Two-year infant health and maternal outcomes, *Nurs Res* 52(2):127-36.

Parker B, McFarlane J, Soeken K, et al. (1993). Physical and emotional abuse in pregnancy: A comparison of adult and teenage women, *Nurs Res* 42(3):173-178.

Plach SK, Stevens PE, Moss VA (2004) Social role experiences of women living with rheumatoid arthritis, *J Family Nurs* 10(1):33-49.

U.S. Department of Health and Human Services: Agency for Healthcare Research and Quality. Accessed July 21, 2005 from http://www.ahcpr.gov//.

U.S. Department of Health and Human Services (1992). *Healthy People 2000: Summary report.* No. PH591–50213, Boston, Jones & Bartlett.

University of Texas Health Science Center at San Antonio: Academic Center for Evidence-Based Nursing. Accessed July 21, 2005 from http://www.acestar.uthscsa.edu/.

Van Cleve L, Bossert E, Beecroft P, et al. (2004). The pain experience of children with leukemia during the first year after diagnosis, *Nurs Res* 53(1):1-10.

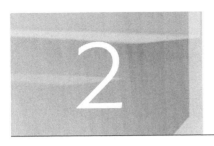

2 The Research Process: Integrating Evidence-Based Practice

INTRODUCTION

Tools are needed for whatever task one sets out to do. Sometimes the tools are relatively simple and concrete (e.g., a pencil). Other times the tools are abstract and more difficult to describe. The tools you need to critically consider research fit into the abstract tool category. They are tools of the mind (e.g., critical thinking and critical reading tools). The following activities are designed to help you recognize and use these tools.

LEARNING OUTCOMES

On completion of this chapter, the student should be able to do the following:

- Identify the steps of quantitative and qualitative research.
- Identify the importance of critical thinking and critical reading for the reading of research articles.
- Identify the steps of critical reading.
- Use the steps of critical reading for reviewing research articles.
- Use identified strategies for critically reading research articles.
- Use identified critical thinking and reading strategies to synthesize critiqued articles.
- Identify components of the levels of evidence.
- Discuss the importance of levels of evidence in relation to being an effective research consumer.
- Identify the format and style of research articles.

Activity 1

Complete each item with the appropriate word or phrase from the text.

1. Critical thinking is a(n) _____ (rational; irrational) process.

2. A noted theorist, Paul (1995) states that critical thinking is a(n) _____ (active; passive), intellectually engaging process in which the reader participates in an _____ (inner; outer) dialogue with the writer.

3. To read critically, readers must enter the point of view of someone other than themselves and instead must enter _____.

4. Nursing students are first introduced to critical thinking skills through utilization of the _____ process of assessment, diagnosis, planning, intervention, and evaluation.

5. What is the minimum number of readings of a research article recommended in the text? _____

Activity 2

Match the term in Column B with the appropriate phrase in Column A. Terms from Column B will be used more than once.

Column A

1. _____ To get a general sense of the material

2. _____ Clarify unfamiliar terms with text

3. _____ Using constructive skepticism

4. _____ Question assumptions

5. _____ Rational examination of ideas

6. _____ Thinking about your own thinking

Column B

a. Critical thinking
b. Critical reading

Activity 3

1. The process of critical reading has four levels, or stages, of understanding. The levels are listed below in a scrambled order. Rearrange the components into the correct order.

   Scrambled order:
   Synthesis understanding
   Preliminary understanding
   Comprehensive understanding
   Analysis understanding

Appropriate order:

a. _____
b. _____
c. _____
d. _____

2. Synthesis understanding, or putting it all together, is one of the final steps in critical reading. It can be broken easily into a series of activities that work best if completed in order. The steps are listed below in a scrambled order; rearrange each set into the appropriate order.

Scrambled order:
Staple the summary to the top of copied article.
Summarize study in your own words.
Complete one handwritten 5 x 8 card per study.
Review your notes on the copy.
Read the article for the fourth time.

Appropriate order:

a. _____
b. _____
c. _____
d. _____
e. _____

Activity 4

Determine whether the article in Appendix D of the text (Davison et al.) is a quantitative or qualitative study. Utilize the following points to determine if the study you are reading is of a quantitative design. First answer *yes* or *no* for each item, then summarize your thoughts in a paragraph.

1. Hypotheses are stated or implied in the article.   Yes   No

2. The terms *control* and *treatment* group appear.   Yes   No

3. The terms *survey, correlational,* or *ex post facto* are used.
   (*Note:* Read the glossary definitions for help in answering
   this question.)   Yes   No

4. The terms *random* or *convenience* are mentioned in
   relation to the sample.   Yes   No

5. Variables are measured by instruments or tools.   Yes   No

6. Reliability and validity of instruments are discussed.   Yes   No

7. Statistical analyses are used.   Yes   No

Summary:

Activity 5

In reading the Plach, Stevens, & Moss (2004) article in Appendix C of the text, you find a reference comparing the differences between mid-life women's and late-life women's emotional well-being: "Despite significantly more health problems, late-life women fared better than their younger counterparts from a psychosocial perspective, reporting more role satisfaction and less depression (Plach, Napholz, & Kelber, 2003a)." You are interested in the reasons for this and believe that you could understand the article better if you could learn more about it. How will you quickly find out about this theory?

Activity 6: Web-Based Activity

Go to the website http://www.criticalthinking.org. Roll your mouse on "About Critical Thinking" at the left and read the following:

*   A Brief History of the Idea of CT
*   Defining Critical Thinking
*   Sumner's Definition of Critical Thinking

    a. Which one of the three articles did you like best?
    b. What did you learn from the article that you liked the best?
    c. List your strengths in critical thinking. Are you open to new experiences and new ways of looking at "problems"? Think about this, and really assess your strengths.
    d. In what areas of critical thinking do you need to improve?

Activity 7: Evidenced-Based Practice Activity

1. Determine the level of evidence for the articles in Appendix B (Van Cleve et al., 2004) and Appendix D (Davison et al., 2003) in your textbook.

2. Find a research article in your area of practice. Determine the level of evidence for the article.

POST-TEST

1. In analyzing research articles it is important to remember that the researcher may _____ (omit; vary) the steps slightly, but that the steps must still be systematically addressed.

2. To critically read a research study, the reader must have skilled reading, writing, and reasoning abilities. Use these abilities to read the following abstract, then identify concepts, clarify any unfamiliar concepts or terms, and question any assumptions or rationales presented.

    This article describes risky drug and sexual behavior and mental health characteristics in a sample of 240 homeless or drug-recovering women and their most immediate sources of social support. … Fifty-one percent of the women and 31% of their support sources had Center for Epidemiological Studies Depression Scale (CES-D) scores of 27 or greater, suggesting a high level of depressive disorders in both samples. Similarly, 76% of the women and 59% of their support sources had psychological well-being scores below a standard clinical cutoff point. These data suggest that homeless and impoverished women turn to individuals who are themselves at high risk for emotional distress and risky behaviors as their main sources of support. (Nyamathi et al., 1997)

    a. Identify concepts.

    b. List any unfamiliar concepts or terms that you would need to clarify.

    c. What assumptions or rationales would you question?

3. Quantitative and qualitative articles will vary a great deal in format and style when they appear in journals. The following statements will focus your attention on these differences and help you to distinguish between the two major types of research. Answer the following questions by inserting the correct term from the list provided. Not all terms will be used.

Used	Conducted
Generate hypotheses	Test a hypothesis
Statistical tests	Analyze themes or concepts

    a. The primary difference between the two is that the qualitative study does not _____ but may _____.
    b. An additional major difference is in the way the literature reviews are _____ and _____ in the study.

Please check with your instructor for the answers to the post-test.

REFERENCES

Davison BJ, Goldenberg SL, Gleave ME, et al. (2003). Provision of individualized information to men and their partners to facilitate treatment decision making in prostate cancer, *Oncol Nurs Forum* 30(1):107-114.

Foundation for Critical Thinking. Accessed July 21, 2005 from http://www.criticalthinking.org.

Nyamathi A, Flaskerud J, Leake B (1997). HIV-risk behaviors and mental health characteristics among homeless or drug-recovering women and their closest sources of social support, *Nurs Res* 46:133-137.

Plach SK, Napholz L, Kelber ST (2003). Depression during early recovery from heart surgery among early middle-age, midlife, and elderly women, *Health Care Women Int* 24:327-339.

Plach SK, Stevens PE, Moss VA (2004) Social role experiences of women living with rheumatoid arthritis, *J Family Nurs* 10(1):33-49.

Van Cleve L, Bossert E, Beecroft P, et al. (2004). The pain experience of children with leukemia during the first year after diagnosis, *Nurs Res* 53(1):1-10.

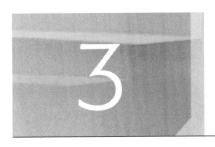

Developing Research Questions and Hypotheses

INTRODUCTION

This chapter focuses on the problem statement and hypothesis. If done correctly, a problem statement can be very helpful to you as a consumer of nursing research because it very concisely (usually in one or two sentences) describes the essence of the research study. For the nurse who considers using the results of a given study in practice, the two primary concerns are to locate the problem statement and critique that problem statement. The hypothesis or the research questions provide the most succinct link between the underlying theoretical base and the research design. Thus, its analysis is pivotal to the analysis of the entire research study.

LEARNING OUTCOMES

On completion of this chapter, the student should be able to do the following:

- Describe how the research question and hypothesis relate to the other components of the research process.
- Describe the process of identifying and refining a research question.
- Identify the criteria for determining the significance of a research question.
- Discuss the purpose of developing a clinical question.
- Identify the characteristics of research questions and hypotheses.
- Discuss the appropriate use of the purpose, aim, or objective of a research study.
- Discuss how the purpose, research question, and hypothesis suggest the level of evidence to be obtained from the findings of a research study.
- Describe the advantages and disadvantages of directional and nondirectional hypotheses.
- Compare and contrast the use of statistical vs. research hypotheses.
- Discuss the appropriate use of research questions vs. hypotheses in a research study.
- Discuss the differences between a research question and a clinical question in relation to evidence-based practice.
- Identify the criteria used for critiquing a research question and hypothesis.
- Apply the critiquing criteria to the evaluation of a research question and hypothesis in a research report.

Activity 1

Match the terms in Column B to the appropriate phrase in Column A. Not all terms from Column B will be used.

Column A

1. _____ An interrogative sentence or declarative statement about the relationship between two or more variables

2. _____ The variable that has the presumed effect on the second variable

3. _____ The variable that is not manipulated

4. _____ A property of the problem that indicates it is measurable by either qualitative or quantitative methods

5. _____ The concepts or properties that are operationalized and studied

Column B

a. Testability
b. Independent variable
c. Variables
d. Dependent variable
e. Problem statement
f. Hypothesis

Activity 2

A good problem statement exhibits four characteristics. Read the problem statements below and examine them to determine if each of the four criteria is present. Following each problem statement is a list representing the four criteria (a-d). Circle *yes* or *no* to indicate whether each criterion is met.

The problem statement:

a. Clearly and unambiguously identifies the variables under consideration
b. Clearly expresses the variables' relationship to each other
c. Specifies the nature of the population being studied
d. Implies the possibility of empirical testing

1. The purpose of this study was to describe the association between the marital relationship and the health of the wife with chronic fatigue and immune dysfunction syndrome (CFIDS). (Goodwin 1997)

    Criterion a: Yes   No

    Criterion b: Yes   No

Criterion c: Yes   No

Criterion d: Yes   No

2. This study examined the effects of an individualized computerized testing system for baccalaureate nursing students enrolled in health assessment and obstetrics/women's health during a 3-year period. (Bloom & Trice 1997)

Criterion a: Yes   No

Criterion b: Yes   No

Criterion c: Yes   No

Criterion d: Yes   No

3. This study was an examination of perceptions about the causes of coronary artery disease and the timeline of the disease among 105 patients hospitalized because of myocardial infarction or for coronary angiography and receiving the diagnosis of coronary artery disease (Zerwic et al. 1997)

Criterion a: Yes   No

Criterion b: Yes   No

Criterion c: Yes   No

Criterion d: Yes   No

Activity 3

The ability to distinguish between independent and dependent variables is a crucial preliminary step to determine whether a research hypothesis is a succinct statement of the relationship between two variables. Identify the variables in the following examples. Decide which is the independent (presumed cause) variable and which is the dependent (presumed effect) variable.

1. The use of cathode ray terminals (CRTs) increases the incidence of birth defects.
    a. Independent variable:

    b. Dependent variable:

2. Individuals with birth defects have a higher incidence of independence-dependence conflicts than individuals without birth defects.
    a. Independent variable:

    b. Dependent variable:

3. What is the relationship between daily moderate consumption of white wine and serum cholesterol levels?
   a. Independent variable:

   b. Dependent variable:

4. Problem-oriented recording leads to more effective patient care than narrative recording.
   a. Independent variable:

   b. Dependent variable:

5. Nurses and physicians differ in the way they view the extended-role concept for nurses.
   a. Independent variable:

   b. Dependent variable:

6. The purpose of this study was to determine the extent to which sex, age, height, and weight predict selected physiologic outcomes; namely, forced expiratory volume in one second (FEV_1), hemoglobin concentration, food intake, serum glucose concentration, total serum cholesterol concentration, and cancer-related weight change. (Brown et al. 1997)
   a. Independent variable:

   b. Dependent variable:

Activity 4

Now take each hypothesis (or research question) from Activity 3 and label it with the appropriate abbreviation from the key provided. More than one abbreviation from the key may be used to describe each item.

Key: RQ = Research question
RP = Research problem
DH = Directional hypothesis
NDH = Nondirectional hypothesis
Hr = Research hypothesis
Ho = Statistical hypothesis

1. _____ The use of cathode ray terminals (CRTs) increases the incidence of birth defects.

2. _____ Individuals with birth defects have a higher incidence of independence-dependence conflicts than individuals without birth defects.

3. _____ What is the relationship between daily moderate consumption of white wine and serum cholesterol levels?

4. _____ Problem-oriented recording leads to more effective patient care than narrative recording.

5. _____ Nurses and physicians differ in the way they view the extended-role concept for nurses.

6. _____ The purpose of this study was to determine the extent to which sex, age, height, and weight predict selected physiologic outcomes, namely, forced expiratory volume in one second (FEV$_1$), hemoglobin concentration, food intake, serum glucose concentration, total serum cholesterol concentration, and cancer-related weight change. (Brown et al. 1997)

Activity 5

The next step is to practice writing hypotheses of different types. Return to the first three of the six hypotheses/questions/problems you labeled in Activity 4. Each was labeled as a specific type of hypothesis, research question, or problem statement. Rewrite each of the first three to meet the conditions of the remaining four types of questions or hypotheses. The first problem is partially completed to provide an example.

1. The use of cathode ray terminals (CRTs) increases the incidence of birth defects.

   DH   *The use of CRTs increases the incidence of birth defects.*

   NDH   *The use of CRTs influences the incidence of birth defects.*

   Hr   *The use of CRTs increases the incidence of birth defects.*

   RQ

   Ho

2. Individuals with birth defects have a higher incidence of independence-dependence conflicts than individuals without birth defects.

   DH

   NDH

   Hr

   RQ

   Ho

3. What is the relationship between daily moderate consumption of white wine and serum cholesterol levels?

   DH

   NDH

   Hr

   RQ

   Ho

Activity 6

Critique the following hypotheses. There were two hypotheses tested in this study.

1. *Hypothesis I:* There will be significant improvement in the dressing independence of cognitively impaired nursing home residents following implementation of strategies to promote independence in dressing (SPID). (Beck et al. 1997)
   a. Is the hypothesis clearly stated in a declarative form?

      Yes   No
   b. Are the independent and dependent variables identified in the statement of the hypothesis?

      Yes   No
   c. Are the variables measurable or potentially measurable?

      Yes   No
   d. Is the hypothesis stated in such a way that it is testable?

      Yes   No
   e. Is the hypothesis stated objectively without value-laden words?

      Yes   No
   f. Is the direction of the relationship in the hypothesis clearly stated?

      Yes   No
   g. Is each of the hypotheses specific to one relationship so that each hypothesis can be either supported or not supported?

      Yes   No

2. *Hypothesis II:* There will be no difference in the time required by nursing assistants to complete dressing activities with cognitively impaired residents before and after implementing strategies to promote independence in dressing (SPID). (Beck et al. 1997)

   a. Is the hypothesis clearly stated in a declarative form?

   Yes   No

   b. Are the independent and dependent variables identified in the statement of the hypothesis?

   Yes   No

   c. Are the variables measurable or potentially measurable?

   Yes   No

   d. Is the hypothesis stated in such a way that it is testable?

   Yes   No

   e. Is the hypothesis stated objectively without value-laden words?

   Yes   No

   f. Is the direction of the relationship in the hypothesis clearly stated?

   Yes   No

   g. Is each of the hypotheses specific to one relationship so that each hypothesis can be either supported or not supported?

   Yes   No

Activity 7

1. You are designing a research study as part of the graduation requirements for your master's degree in nursing. In your personal timeline, you have committed 1 year (two 15-week semesters) to designing, obtaining human subjects approval, data collection, analysis, writing, and conducting the oral defense of this master's thesis. You would like to study the effect on patient outcomes on a cardiac unit based on the introduction of patient care technicians as team members to replace the primary care nursing model. The feasibility issues you will need to consider are time, availability of subjects, money, facilities and equipment, experience of the researcher, and ethical issues. For each of these issues described above, give your considered opinion as to why this study would or would not be feasible.

   a. Time
   b. Availability of subjects, money, facilities, and equipment
   c. Experience of the researcher
   d. Ethical issues

2. Another important element to consider when deciding to conduct research is to determine if this is a significant enough topic to study. Would the outcomes study proposed meet the criteria to be considered significant? Answer *yes* or *no* and then give the rationale underlying your choice.

Activity 8

How do you determine whether a sentence is a problem statement or a hypothesis? Please explain.

Activity 9: Web-Based Activity

1. Go to the website http://www.socialresearchmethods.net/kb/probform.htm. Read "Problem Formulation."

2. Go to the website http://www.nursing-standard.co.uk/archives/ns/vol13-27/research.htm. Read "Historical research: process, problems and pitfalls."

3. Go to the website http://www.ahrq.gov/. Click on "AHRQ Research Agenda" under Funding Opportunities. Are any of the listed research agenda items of interest to you?

Activity 10: Evidence-Based Practice Activity

1. Develop a research question in an area of nursing practice that is of interest to you.

2. Identify the independent and dependant variables.

3. Identify the population.

POST-TEST

1. Choose the terms from the key provided that best describe items a through h. Write the appropriate abbreviation in the space provided. More than one abbreviation from the key may be used to describe each item.

Key: RQ = Research question
DH = Directional hypothesis
NDH = Nondirectional hypothesis
Hr = Research hypothesis
Ho = Statistical hypothesis

a. _____ There will be no change in self-rated body image among women in the three patient groups.

b. _____ What is the relationship between organizational climate dimensions and job satisfaction of nurses in neonatal intensive care units?

c. _____ The higher the perceived parental support, the lower the girls' general fearfulness.

d. _____ There will be a significant difference in pre/post changes in cognitive development level between undergraduate nursing students who have completed a research course and those who have not.

e. _____ The post-test mean of selected psychological variables for the experimental group will be lower than that of the control group.

f. _____ There will be no association found between the level of social support and self-care health practices.

g. _____ The educational preparation of a nurse (e.g., AA, diploma, BS) will affect his/her ability to conduct thorough patient interviews.

h. _____ What is the level of postoperative infection following the use of clean tracheotomy care?

2. Fill in the blanks in the following sentences with the appropriate word or words from the list provided. Not all the words in the list will be used.

Research	Null
Predicts	Validity
Statistical	Directional
Testing	Declarative statement
Nondirectional	Research question

a. The hypothesis is a vehicle for _____ the _____ of the assumptions of the theoretical framework of a research study.

b. A hypothesis transposes the question posed by the research problem into a _____ that _____ the relationship between two or more variables.

c. _____ hypotheses are more common than _____ hypotheses in studies that utilize deductive reasoning.

d. A _____ hypothesis is also known as the _____ hypothesis.

3. Refer to the Plach et al. (2004) article in Appendix C of the text.
    a. Highlight the problem statement or hypothesis.
    b. Is it a <u>problem statement</u> or <u>hypothesis</u>? (Circle the correct answer.)
    c. List the variables being studied.

    d. Critique the problem statement or hypothesis in the article focusing on the four criteria listed below. Circle your answers.

        Criterion a: Clearly and unambiguously identifies the variables under consideration

        Yes   No

        Criterion b: Clearly expresses the variables' relationship to each other

        Yes   No

        Criteria c: Specifies the nature of the population being studied

        Yes   No

        Criterion d: Implies the possibility of empirical testing

        Yes   No

    e. Has the problem been placed within the context of an appropriate theoretical framework? If the answer is yes, list the framework described in the study.

4. Refer to the Davison et al. (2003) article in Appendix D of the text.
    a. Highlight the problem statement or hypothesis.
    b. Is it a <u>problem statement</u> or <u>hypothesis</u>? (Circle the correct answer.)
    c. List the variables being studied:

    d. Critique the problem statement or hypothesis in the article focusing on the four criteria listed below. Circle the correct answers.

        Criterion a: Clearly and unambiguously identifies the variables under consideration

        Yes   No

        Criterion b: Clearly expresses the variables' relationship to each other

        Yes   No

        Criterion c: Specifies the nature of the population being studied

        Yes   No

Criterion d: Implies the possibility of empirical testing

Yes   No

e. Has the problem been placed within the context of an appropriate theoretical frame-work? If the answer is yes, list the framework described in the study.

Please check with your instructor for the answer to the post-test.

REFERENCES

Beck C et al. (1997). Improving dressing behavior in cognitively impaired nursing home residents, *Nurs Res* 46:126–131.

Bloom K, Trice L (1997). The efficacy of individualized computerized testing in nursing education, *Computer Nurs* 15:82–88.

Brown J, Knapp T, Radke K (1997). Sex, age, height, and weight as predictors of selected physiologic outcomes, *Nurs Res* 46:101–104.

Davison BJ, Goldenberg SL, Gleave ME, et al. (2003). Provision of individualized information to men and their partners to facilitate treatment decision making in prostate cancer, *Oncol Nurs Forum* 30(1):107–114.

Goodwin S (1997). The marital relationship and health in women with chronic fatigue and immune dysfunction syndrome: Views of wives and husbands, *Nurs Res* 46:138–146.

Plach SK, Stevens PE, Moss VA (2004) Social role experiences of women living with rheumatoid arthritis, *J Family Nurs* 10(1):33–49.

Rees C, Howells G (1999). Historical research: Process, problems and pitfalls. *Nurs Stand* 13, 27, 33–35. Accessed July 22, 2005 from http://www.nursing-standard.co.uk/archives/ns/vol13-27/research.htm.

Trochim WMK: Research methods knowledge base: Problem formulation. Accessed July 22, 2005 from http://www.socialresearchmethods.net/kb/probform.htm.

U.S. Department of Health and Human Services: Agency for Healthcare Research and Quality. Accessed July 21, 2005 from http://www.ahrq.gov/.

Zerwic JJ, King KB, Wlasowicz GS (1997). Perceptions of patients with cardiovascular disease about the causes of coronary artery disease, *Heart Lung* 26:92–98.

Literature Review

INTRODUCTION

The most common usage of the term *review of the literature* is to refer to that section of a research study in which the researcher describes the linkage between previously existing knowledge and the current study. Other research-related uses of a review of the literature are as follows:

1. Developing an overall impression of what research and clinical work has been done in a given area
2. Assisting in the clarification of the research problem
3. Polishing research design ideas
4. Finding possible data collection and data analysis strategies

This chapter will help you learn more about each of these uses of the literature to provide you with the basic information needed to decide whether a researcher has thoroughly reviewed the relevant literature, and used this review to its fullest potential.

LEARNING OUTCOMES

On completion of this chapter, the student should be able to do the following:

- Discuss the relationship of the literature review to nursing theory, research, education, and practice.
- Discuss the purposes of the literature review from the perspective of the research investigator and the research consumer.
- Discuss the use of the literature review for quantitative designs and qualitative approaches.
- Discuss the purpose of reviewing the literature in development of evidence-based practice.
- Differentiate between conceptual (theoretical) and data-based (research literature).
- Differentiate between primary and secondary sources.

- Compare the advantages and disadvantages of the most commonly used online databases and print database sources for conducting a literature review.
- Identify the characteristics of a relevant literature review.
- Differentiate between a study's literature review and a systematic review.
- Differentiate between a qualitative systematic review and a quantitative systematic review (meta-analysis).
- Critically read, critique, and synthesize conceptual and data-based resources for the development of a literature review.
- Apply critiquing criteria to the evaluation of literature reviews in selected research studies.

Activity 1

In the sentences listed below, fill in the blanks with the appropriate word or words from the italicized terms found in the following sentence:

The review of the literature is essential to the growth of nursing *theory, research, education,* and *practice.* In relation to these four concepts, a critical review of the literature does the following:

1. Reveals appropriate _____ questions for the discipline.

2. Provides the latest knowledge for _____ .

3. Uncovers _____ findings that can lead to changes in clinical
   _____ .

4. Uncovers new knowledge that can lead to the refinement of _____ .

Activity 2

Listed below are examples of uses of the literature for research consumer purposes in educational and practice settings. Match the title of the research consumer in Column B with the description of activities in Column A. The titles will be used more than once.

Column A – Activities

1. _____ Develop ANA's social policy statement
2. _____ Implement research-based nursing interventions
3. _____ Develop scholarly academic papers
4. _____ Develop AHRQ's practice guidelines
5. _____ Develop research proposals for master's thesis
6. _____ Evaluate hospital CQI programs
7. _____ Revise curricula

Column B – Titles

a. Undergraduate student
b. Faculty
c. Nurses in clinical setting
d. Graduate students
e. Governmental agencies
f. Professional nursing organizations

Activity 3

Following is a list of terms and examples describing either conceptual or data-based literature. Put a *C* if the example describes conceptual literature, or a *D* if the example describes data-based literature. Refer to Tables 4-4 and 4-7 of the text for help.

1. _____ Published quantitative and qualitative studies
2. _____ Published articles or books discussing theories or concepts
3. _____ Unpublished abstracts of research studies from research conference
4. _____ Published studies in journal describing relationships between variables
5. _____ Teel C et al. (1997). Perspectives unifying symptom interpretation, *Image: J Nurs Schol* 29:175–181. The purpose was to introduce the symptom interpretation model (SIM) and facilitate understanding symptoms from an intrapersonal perspective. Theory derivation was used to develop SIM for understanding comparisons of known and new symptoms in a behavioral outcomes context.
6. _____ Oldham J, Howe T (1997). The effectiveness of placebo muscle stimulation in quadriceps muscle rehabilitation: A preliminary evaluation, *Clin Effectiv Nurs* 1:25–30. The objective of this study was to evaluate the effect of placebo and "active" muscle stimulation in the rehabilitation of quadriceps muscle function in patients with osteoarthritis of the knee. All subjects were recruited from a waiting list for knee joint replacement.

Activity 4

Researchers who are also clinicians are interested in solving clinical problems—whether the solution is for immediate or future use. When faced with a problem in clinical practice, a clinician's common first thought is: What have others learned about this problem? The clinician usually goes first to the nursing literature to seek an answer to that question. List *five* nursing journals that publish reports or research studies that you as a clinician might study to find out more about a problem.

1. _____

2. _____

3. _____

4. _____

5. _____

Activity 5

The review of the literature is *usually* easy to find. In the abridged version of a research report, it is clearly labeled. Most frequently, one of the early sections of the report is labeled *Review of Literature* or *Relevant Literature* or some other comparable term. It may also be separated into a literature review section, and another section entitled *Conceptual Framework* that presents material on the theoretical or conceptual framework, which serves as the foundation for the study.

1. Examine the first two articles that are in the appendices of the text. What title is given to the literature review section?
    a. In Koniak-Griffin et al.:

    b. In Van Cleve et al.:

(*Note:* The length of the literature review section in a journal varies. A range from two paragraphs to several paragraphs is the most common.)

2. Does the literature review uncover gaps or inconsistencies in knowledge? If yes, state in your own words what gap or inconsistency is identified. If no, simply write "No."
    a. In Koniak-Griffin et al.:

    b. In Van Cleve et al.:

3. Return to the Koniak-Griffin et al. article. Determine how recent the articles listed in the reference section are. There should be some from within 3 to 5 years and they should portray the development of the research over time. It should read like a good detective story, where at first there may be qualitative studies that attempt to identify which variables are important to this problem or paradigm. At some point you should also see researchers progressively analyze each of the variables, gradually narrowing and defining the scope of the problem, while others continue to look at the problem qualitatively. Do you see this in the literature and reference section of the Koniak-Griffin et al. article?   Yes   No

Critique the currency of the references. Write the story you see in the reference section and as described in the review of the literature.

Activity 6

Sometimes it is difficult to understand the distinction between primary and secondary sources of information. A comparison that is always helpful is if you are considering giving a client an injection for pain, whose report would you feel most comfortable evaluating—the report of a family member or nurse's aide (i.e., secondary source) or the report by the client (i.e., primary source)? As a consumer of nursing research, you will also need to evaluate the credibility of research designs and reports based in part on whether they are generated from primary or secondary sources so that you know whether the information you are reading is a first-hand report or someone else's interpretation of the material.

1. The following words or phrases describe either primary or secondary sources. Put a *P* next to those describing primary sources, and an *S* next to those describing secondary sources.

    a. _____ Summaries of research studies

    b. _____ First-hand accounts

    c. _____ Biographies

    d. _____ Textbooks

    e. _____ Patient records

    f. _____ Reports written by the researcher

    g. _____ Dissertations or master's theses

2. The best source for primary research studies is the World Wide Web.   True   False

3. You have a computer with a fast modem, web access provider, and web browser service at your home. You can now do your literature search in CINAHL OnLine without any additional cost.

    True   False

4. Information about CINAHL products and links to other nursing sources can be accessed at http://www.cinahl.com/.

    True   False

5. Which is the best database for a search of nursing literature?
    a. MEDLINE
    b. CINAHL

    Why is one better than the other for nursing literature?

6. Print databases, such as CINAHL Print Index, must be used for literature searches of material before 1982.

    True   False

7. There is usually an extra charge for full text access to an article by fax or modem over the Internet from CINAHL (http://www.cinahl.com/) or another provider, such as Medical Matrix (http://www.medmatrix.org/info/medlinetable.html).

    True   False

8. The Sigma Theta Tau Law Registry of Nursing Research (http://www.stti.org/VirginiaHendersonLibrary/) and the Online Journal of Knowledge Synthesis for Nursing are available on the web for free.

    True   False

Activity 7

Below is a selected list of references from the Koniak-Griffin et al. article (Appendix A in the textbook). Next to each, indicate whether the reference is conceptual (*C*) or data-based (*D*), and whether it is primary (*P*) or secondary (*S*). Sometimes it is helpful to return to the text of the article and read the discussion of the reference; this may quickly inform you of the type of article that is referenced.

1. _____ _____ Chausen JA (1991). Adolescent competence and the life course, or why one social psychologist needed a concept of personality, *Soc Psychol Q* 54:4-14.

2. _____ _____ Kitzman H, Olds DL, Henderson CR, et al. (1997). Effect of prenatal and infancy home visitation by nurses on pregnancy outcomes, childhood injuries, and repeated childbearing: A randomized clinical trial, *JAMA* 278:644-652.

3. _____ _____ Koniak-Griffin D, Anderson NIR, Verzemnieks I, et al. (2000). A public health nursing early intervention program for adolescent mothers: Outcomes from pregnancy through 6 weeks postpartum, *Nurs Res* 49:130-138.

4. _____ _____ Marin G, Marin BV, *Research with Hispanic Populations* (Vol. 23) Applied Social Research Methods Series, Newbury Park, CA, 1991: Sage.

5. _____ _____ Olds DI, Eckenrode J, Henderson CR, et al. (1997). Long-term effects of home visitation on maternal life course and child abuse and neglect: Fifteen-year follow-up of a randomized trial, *JAMA* 278:637-643.

Activity 8

Many health care professionals and consumers now use the Internet to search for health care information. Before going on the Internet, develop a set of questions that you would like to use to critique the scientific merit of health care information obtained from the Internet. List at least *five* questions.

It may be helpful to recall what you have learned about the peer-review process before journal articles are accepted for publication, and to review the critiquing criteria in the textbook.

1.

2.

3.

4.

5.

Activity 9: Web-Based Activity

1. Go to the website http://www.cinahl.com and explore the site. How much does it cost to sign up for service?

2. Go to the website http://www.ncbi.nlm.nih.gov/entrez/query.fcgi and work through the tutorial on PubMed.

Activity 10: Evidence-Based Practice Activity

1. Do a literature search for the question that you developed in chapter 3.

2. How many total articles did you find related to your question?

3. How many research articles did you find related to your question?

4. For each article, indicate whether it is conceptual or data-based, and whether it is primary or secondary.

POST-TEST

1. Indicate whether the following are examples of primary (*P*) or secondary (*S*) sources.
   a. _____ Pell J (1997). Cardiac rehabilitation: A review of its effectiveness, *Cor Health Care* 1:8–17. This article reviews the published literature on the effectiveness of cardiac rehabilitation in terms of improving mortality, quality of life, and employment in those with myocardial infarction and stable angina pectoris.
   b. _____ Zalon M (1997). Pain in frail, elderly women after surgery, *Image: J Nurs Schol* 29:21–26. The purpose was to describe the lived experience of postoperative pain in frail, elderly women using Colaizzi's (1978) phenomenological approach.

2. Turn to the reference section in the Davison BJ et al. article (Appendix D in the textbook), which is partially reproduced below. Next to each reference indicate whether it is conceptual (*C*), or data-based (*D*), and whether it is primary (*P*), or secondary (*S*).
   a. _____ _____ Beisecker AE, Moore WP (1994). Oncologists' perceptions of the effects of cancer patients: Companions on physician-patient interactions, *J Psychosocial Oncol* 12(1/2):23-39.
   b. _____ _____ Cohen R, Lazarus RD (1979). In Stone GC, Cohen F, Adler NF, eds., Coping with stress of illness, *Health Psychology*, San Francisco: Jossey-Bass, 217-224.
   c. _____ _____ Davison BJ, Degner IF, Morgan TR (1995). Information and decision-making preferences of men with prostate cancer, *Oncol Nurs Forum* 22:1401-1408.
   d. _____ _____ Moore KN, Estey A (1999). The early post-operative concerns of men after radical prostatectomy, *J Adv Nurs* 29:1121-1129.

3. Fill in the correct term.

a. There are many _____ (advantages; disadvantages) for using computer databases rather than just print databases when doing a literature search.

b. _____ (Primary; Secondary) sources are essential for literature reviews when designing a research proposal.

c. The consumer of research should acquire the ability to _____ (critically evaluate a review of the literature using critiquing criteria; use primary and secondary sources to write a literature review for a research study).

d. To efficiently retrieve scholarly literature the nurse must both consult the reference librarian and _____ (independently use e-mail; use computer CINAHL CD-ROM databases).

Please check with your instructor for the answers to the post-test.

REFERENCES

Beisecker AE, Moore WP (1994). Oncologists' perceptions of the effects of cancer patients: Companions on physician-patient interactions, *J Psychosocial Oncol* 12(1/2):23-39.

Chausen JA (1991). Adolescent competence and the life course, or why one social psychologist needed a concept of personality, *Soc Psychol Q* 54:4-14.

CINAHL Information Systems. Accessed July 21, 2005 from http://www.cinahl.com.

Cohen R, Lazarus RD (1979). In Stone GC, Cohen F, Adler NF, eds., Coping with stress of illness, *Health Psychology,* San Francisco: Jossey-Bass, 217-224.

Davison BJ, Goldenberg SL, Gleave ME, et al. (2003). Provision of individualized information to men and their partners to facilitate treatment decision making in prostate cancer, *Oncol Nurs Forum* 30(1):107-114.

Davison BJ, Degner IF, Morgan TR (1995). Information and decision-making preferences of men with prostate cancer, *Oncol Nurs Forum* 22:1401-1408.

Kitzman H, Olds DL, Henderson CR, et al. (1997). Effect of prenatal and infancy home visitation by nurses on pregnancy outcomes, childhood injuries, and repeated childbearing: A randomized clinical trial, *JAMA* 278:644-652.

Koniak-Griffin D, Anderson NIR, Verzemnieks I, et al. (2000). A public health nursing early intervention program for adolescent mothers: Outcomes from pregnancy through 6 weeks postpartum, *Nurs Res* 49:130-138.

Koniak-Griffin D, Verzemnieks IL, Anderson NLR, et al. (2003). Nurse visitation for adolescent mothers: Two-year infant health and maternal outcomes, *Nurs Res* 52(2):127-136.

Marin G, Marin BV (1991). *Research with Hispanic Populations* (Vol. 23), Applied Social Research Methods Series, Newbury Park, CA: Sage.

Moore KN, Estey A (1999). The early post-operative concerns of men after radical prostatectomy, *J Adv Nurs* 29:1121-1129.

Oldham J, Howe T (1997). The effectiveness of placebo muscle stimulation in quadriceps muscle rehabilitation: a preliminary evaluation, *Clin Effectiv Nurs* 1:25-30.

Olds DI, Eckenrode J, Henderson CR, et al. (1997). Long-term effects of home visitation on maternal life course and child abuse and neglect: Fifteen-year follow-up of a randomized trial, *JAMA* 278:637-643.

Pell J (1997). Cardiac rehabilitation: A review of its effectiveness, *Cor Health Care* 1:8-17.

Sigma Theta Tau International: Virginia Henderson International Nursing Library. Accessed July 21, 2005 from http://www.stti.org/VirginiaHendersonLibrary/.

Teel C et al. (1997). Perspectives unifying symptom interpretation, *Image: J Nurs Schol* 29:175-181.

Van Cleve L, Bossert E, Beecroft P, et al. (2004). The pain experience of children with leukemia during the first year after diagnosis, *Nurs Res* 53(1):1-10.

Zalon M (1997). Pain in frail, elderly women after surgery, *Image: J Nurs Schol* 29:21-26.

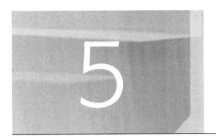

Theoretical Framework

INTRODUCTION

It is not uncommon for the beginning consumer of research to find the theoretical part of a study to be the least favorite component. It tends to be heavily documented and is slow reading. It will not be long before you find it to be a very valuable aspect of any study. The theoretical framework of a study provides you with the opportunity to see the research problem through the eyes of the researcher. As the researcher develops and writes this section of the study, a window to his or her mind is opened. You get a glimpse of the way this particular researcher thinks about this particular problem. A critiquer's task is to listen respectfully to that person's perspective and then ask the following questions:

- How clearly do I understand the researcher's argument?
- Does the theoretical framework connect all of the pieces of the study?
- Can I see the relationship between the theoretical discussion and my clinical practice?

Most of the exercises in this chapter address the first question. Your ability to answer the second and third questions will improve as you complete the research course and as you build your clinical experiences.

LEARNING OBJECTIVES

On completion of this chapter, the student should be able to do the following:

- Compare inductive and deductive reasoning.
- Differentiate between conceptual and theoretical frameworks.
- Identify the purpose and nature of conceptual and theoretical frameworks.
- Describe how a framework guides research.
- Differentiate between conceptual and operational definitions.
- Describe the relationship between theory and research and practice.
- Discuss levels of abstraction related to frameworks guiding research.
- Differentiate among grand, midrange, and microrange theories in nursing.

• Describe the points of critical appraisal used to evaluate the appropriateness, cohesiveness, and consistency of a framework guiding research.

Activity 1

1. Jot down in your own words the defining characteristics of:

   Inductive thinking:

   Deductive thinking:

2. Play with these two kinds of thinking (inductive and deductive thinking) a bit before moving to clinical examples.

   a. Imagine you are hungry. You look around for something to eat. You find a decorative tin labeled "candy" and decide that sounds good. You open the tin and see what looks like multicolored oval beads. It sure does not look like any candy you have ever seen before, but you trust the person who would be putting things in this tin, so you decide to try them. Before long you notice yourself looking for the mottled pink, orange, yellow, and black ones because these taste good. You leave the mottled yellow, white, and reddish-brown ones alone because you do not like them.

      (Inductive; Deductive) _____ thinking would best describe your activity.

   b. Some time later you feel those old hunger pangs returning. This time the candy tin is empty. You want some more of those sweet multicolored oval beads. You start thinking, "Those beads were in the candy tin. They were sweet. There is a candy store around the corner. I bet the candy store will have these sweet beads. You walk to the candy store and discover that your thinking was correct. The candy store does have those sweet beads, and they call them jelly beans.

      (Inductive; Deductive) _____ describes your thinking style in this situation.

3. Now think about the concept of "pain." Think even more specifically about "headache pain." Picture several individuals, including yourself, when they are experiencing a headache. List your observations.

   Person #1   **Person #2**   **Person #3**   **Person #4**

Look across those observations. See any similarities? Maybe a creased forehead? Rubbing temples with fingertips? Rubbing forehead? Rubbing back of neck? Grumpy? Prefer less light? Reach for the over-the-counter pain medication? Grimaces?

Could you write a general statement about "signs of headache pain"? If yes, please do so; if no, jot down your thinking about why you are unable to write such a general statement.

Activity 2

As explained in the text, concepts are the building blocks of a study. The greater the ease with which you can identify concepts the easier it will become to analyze the theoretical framework of a given study. Once you can perform this analysis, you will be able to follow the line of logic from problem to conclusions.

1. Identify the concepts in each of the following excerpts from research:

   a. "A theoretical model was developed and tested to explain the effects of learned help-lessness, self-esteem, and depression on the health practices of homeless women." (Flynn, 1997)

   b. "… was to examine the relationships among illness, uncertainty, stress, coping, and emotional well-being at the time of entry into a clinical drug trial" (Wineman et al., 1996)

   c. "As part of a larger study of the impact of a social support intervention on pregnancy outcome for lower-income African-American women …" (Bolla et al., 1996)

   d. "… to identify determinants of violent and nonviolent behavior among a group of vulnerable inner-city youths." (Powell, 1997)

   e. "… prevalence and consequences of verbal abuse of staff nurses by physicians were examined in the context of Lazarus' stress-coping model." (Manderino and Berkey, 1997)

2. Now let's make things a bit more complex. Remember the definition of a *concept*? Sure you do! It is an abstraction. It is a term that creates an image of an idea or some notion that we humans want to share. Some concepts are more abstract than others. For example, "love" is more abstract than "table." Frequently, the terms *concept* and *construct* are used interchangeably. There is a subtle difference.

    a. Which term (beauty or nursing diagnosis) is a concept? Which is a construct?

    b. Think about the concept and construct in the previous question. How are they alike?

    c. How are they different?

3. Now it is your turn. Choose one concept from each of the five research examples in Item #1 of this activity. Write a definition of the chosen concept. Use your own words.

    a.

    b.

    c.

    d.

    e.

4. Compare your definition of the chosen concept with the definition of the same concept written by one of your peers. How close were you? Think about those similarities and differences. Assume the two of you were going to work as co-investigators on a study that addressed the chosen concept.

    a. What would you need to resolve?

    b. Look one more time at those concepts. Do any of them more closely resemble a construct?

Activity 3

You have identified concepts, and you have written a definition of a concept. It is highly probable that the definition you wrote had more in common with a conceptual definition than with an operational definition. Operational definitions are a bit trickier. They need to be so clear that you, the reader, have no questions about what the researcher meant by each concept.

Think about the concept of "verbal abuse." What comes to mind when you hear that term (e.g., specific words such as swearing, put-downs, sarcasm; tone of voice, loudness of voice, frequency of abuse)? Verbal abuse was defined by Manderino and Berkey (1997) as the score on "the Verbal Abuse Scale (VAS)." They go on to explain that the Verbal Abuse Scale is "a recently developed 65-item self-report questionnaire, clearly defining 11 different forms of verbal abuse, thus permitting a focused exploration of the frequency and perceived stressfulness of the various manifestations of abuse." The 11 categories of verbal abuse are: ignoring, abusive anger, condescending, blocking/diverting, trivializing, abuse disguised as a joke, accusing/blaming, judging/criticizing, sexual harassment, discounting, and threatening. Turn to the studies included in the four appendices of the textbook. Identify the conceptual and operational definitions in each of these studies. Do not expect every study to include both, and do not be surprised if some definitions are implicit rather than explicit.

1. Koniak-Griffin, et al.:

2. Van Cleve, et al.:

3. Plach, Stevens, & Moss:

4. Davison, et al.:

Activity 4

Let's take a quick look at how theory, concepts, definitions, variables, and hypotheses fit together. There will be more detail about variables and hypotheses in a later chapter, so the focus here is more on an understanding of how they are based in theory.

1. Match the terms in Column B with the appropriate definition or example in Column A. Words in **bold** print in Column A indicate the element to be matched to a term. Items in Column B may be used more than once.

Column A

a. _____ "Fatigue symptoms were measured using the Modified Fatigue Symptoms Checklist (MFSC), a list of 30 symptoms of fatigue. Scores range from zero (no fatigue symptoms) to 30 symptoms (maximum fatigue)." (Milligan, Flenniken, and Pugh, 1996)

b. _____ "… **stress** and **empowerment** were used to guide this study." (Kendra, 1996)

c. _____ "Serenity is viewed as a learned, positive emotion of inner peace that can be sustained … that decreases perceived stress and improves physical and emotional health." (Roberts and Whall, 1996)

d. _____ Older (i.e., **more than 35 years old**) first-time mothers (Reese and Harkless, 1996)

e. _____ Clinical decision-making

f. _____ Quality of life

g. _____ "Acute confusion is a transient syndrome characterized primarily by abnormalities in attention and cognition, but disordered psychomotor behavior, sleep-wake disturbance, and autonomic nervous system disturbances are not uncommon." (Neelon et al. 1996)

h. _____ "Are there **breathing pattern changes** from test to test or from the beginning to the end of the test?" (Hopp et al. 1996)

i. _____ "The combination of injury experience, knowledge, demographic, health beliefs, and social influence variables will predict home hazard accessibility." (Russell and Champion, 1996)

Column B
1. Variable
2. Hypothesis
3. Construct
4. Operational definition
5. Concept
6. Conceptual definition

2. This exercise allows you the opportunity to use all of the thinking you have done so far in tracing a variable from the introduction of a study through the theoretical rationale of that same study. Turn to Appendix C of the text and read the first part of the Plach, Stevens, & Moss study. Read from the beginning of the study (including the title) to the section entitled "Method." Do not read the methods section.

    a. Name the main variable in this study (read the title closely for this information):

    b. Read the next six paragraphs and summarize in one sentence per paragraph what you learned about anger.

        i.

        ii.

        iii.

        iv.

        v.

        vi.

    c. What type of reasoning is operating in this study?

    d. Were hypotheses developed for this study?

    e. Would you describe the theoretical rationale for this study as:

        _____ A theoretical framework   _____ A theory

        _____ A conceptual model   _____ None of the above

Activity 5

Use the grid that follows and critique the theoretical component of the four studies found in the appendices of the text. In the grid, identify the study that satisfies that particular criterion, that is, use *K* for Koniak-Griffin et al., *V* for Van Cleve et al., *P* for Plach, Stevens, & Moss, and *D* for Davison et al.

CRITIQUING GRID

	Well Done	OK	Needs Help	Not Applicable
1. Theoretical rationale was clearly identi-fied (Could I find it?)				
2. The information in the theoretical com-ponent matches what the researchers are studying				
3. Concepts:				
a. Conceptual definition(s) found				
b. Conceptual definition(s) clear				
c. Operational definition(s) found				
d. Operational definition(s) clear				
4. Enough literature was reviewed:				
a. For an expert in the area				
b. For a nurse with some knowledge				
c. For a nurse reading outside of area of specialty or interest				
5. Thinking of researcher:				
a. Can be followed through theoretical material to hypotheses or questions				
b. Makes sense				
6. Relationships among propositions clearly stated				
7. Theory:				
a. Borrowed				
b. Concepts/data related to nursing				
8. Findings related back to theoretical base (I can find each concept from the theory section discussed in the "Results" section of the report.)				

Activity 6: Web-Based Activity

Go to the website: http://www.jcu.edu.au/soc/nursoc/html_pages/nursing_research.htm. Go to #7 Conceptual Theoretical Frameworks and explore the conceptual frameworks presented.

Go to the website: http://www.training.nih.gov/student/srfp/catalog/ninr.asp. Identify the conceptual or theoretical framework for each of the research laboratories listed.

POST-TEST

1. List three reasons supporting the importance of the theoretical rationale of a study.

   a.

   b.

   c.

2. Read each statement. Decide if the statement is true or false by marking with a *T* if the statement is true, and with an *F* if the statement is false. Rewrite the false statements to make them true statements.

   a. _____ "Caregiving" is an example of a concept that is so clearly understood there is no need for it to be operationally defined in a research study.

   b. _____ The following definition is an example of a conceptual definition: "The Beck Dressing Performance Scale (BDPS) (Beck, 1988) was used to measure the major dependent variable, the level of caregiver assistance provided during dressing. The dressing function is broken down into 42 discrete component steps for males and 45 for females. A trained rater assigns each step of the dressing activity a score of 0 (independent) to 7 (complete dependence) based on the amount of assistance required to complete each step. Higher scores indicate greater dependence." (Beck et al., 1997)

   c. _____ The words in **bold** in the following phrase are the name of a construct: "… define **a professional practice model** (PPM) as a system that supports registered nurse control over the delivery of nursing care and the environment in which care is delivered." (Hoffart and Woods, 1997)

   d. _____ The following is an example of a conceptual definition: "Although there is no standard definition of social support, there seems to be general acceptance of some basic typologies. House, Umberson, and Landis (1988) defined social support as positive dimensions of relationships that may promote health and buffer stress." (Bolla et al., 1996)

e.   _____   The following is a sketch of a concept: "… verbal abuse was defined as verbal behaviors that are perceived as humiliating, degrading, and/or disrespectful. Because verbally abusive encounters potentially can be stressful, it seemed appropriate to address this issue within the framework of a model of stress … the major tenet of this model [sic: Lazarus' transactional model of stress coping] is that stress occurs in the face of perceived demands that tax or exceed the perceived coping resources of the person." (Manderino and Berkey, 1997)

Please check with your instructor for the answers to the post-test.

REFERENCES

Beck C et al. (1997). Improving dressing behavior in cognitively impaired nursing home residents, *Nurs Res* 46(3):126–132.

Bolla CD et al. (1996). Social support as a road map and vehicle: An analysis of data from focus group interviews with a group of African American women, *Public Health Nurs* 13(5):331–336.

Davison BJ, Goldenberg SL, Gleave ME, et al. (2003). Provision of individualized information to men and their partners to facilitate treatment decision making in prostate cancer, *Oncol Nurs Forum* 30(1):107-114.

Flynn L (1997). The health practices of homeless women: A causal model, *Nurs Res* 46(2): 72–77.

Hoffart N, Woods CQ (1997). Elements of a nursing professional practice model, *J Prof Nurs* 12(6):354–364.

Hopp LJ et al. (1996). Incremental threshold loading in patients with chronic obstructive pulmonary disease, *Nurs Res* 45(4):196–202.

Kendra MA (1996). Perception of risk by home health care administrators and field workers, *Public Health Nurs* 13(6):386–393.

Koniak-Griffin D, Verzemnieks IL, Anderson NLR, et al. (2003). Nurse visitation for adolescent mothers: Two-year infant health and maternal outcomes, *Nurs Res* 52(2):127-136.

Manderino MA, Berkey N (1997). Verbal abuse of staff nurses by physicians, *J Prof Nurs* 13(1): 48–55.

Milligan RA, Flenniken PM, Pugh LC (1996). Positioning intervention to minimize fatigue in breast-feeding women, *Appl Nurs Res* 9(2):67–70.

National Institutes of Health: Research and Training Opportunities. Accessed July 21, 2005 from http://www.training.nih.gov/student/srfp/catalog/ninr.asp.

Neelon VJ et al. (1996). The Neecham confusion scale: Construction, validation, and clinical testing, *Nurs Res* 45(6):324–330.

NURSOC. Accessed July 21, 2005 from http://www.jcu.edu.au/soc/nursoc/html_pages/nursing_research.htm.

Plach SK, Stevens PE, Moss VA (2004). Social role experiences of women living with rheumatoid arthritis, *J Family Nurs* 10(1):33-49.

Powell KB (1997). Correlates of violent and nonviolent behavior among vulnerable inner-city youths, *Family Comm Health* 20(2):38–47.

Reese SM, Harkless G (1996). Clinical methods: Divergent themes in maternal experience in women older than 35 years of age, *Appl Nurs Res* 9(3):148–153.

Roberts KT, Whall A (1996). Serenity as a goal for nursing practice, *Image: J Nurs Schol* 28(4): 359–364.

Russell KM, Champion VL: Health beliefs and social influence in home safety practice of mothers with preschool children, *Image: J Nurs Schol* 28(1):59–64, 1996.

Van Cleve L, Bossert E, Beecroft P, et al. (2004). The pain experience of children with leukemia during the first year after diagnosis, *Nurs Res* 53(1):1-10.

Wineman NM et al. (1996). Relationships among illness uncertainty, stress, coping, and emotional well-being at entry into a clinical drug trial, *Appl Nurs Res* 9(2):53–60.

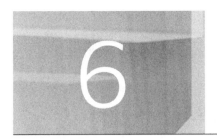

Introduction to Qualitative Research

INTRODUCTION

Using scientific methods is important for solving nursing problems. Although knowledge acquisition comes in a variety of ways, finding the optimal ways to answer nursing questions usually entails research. As nurses, we have a variety of assumptions and beliefs that influence the ways we see and interpret meanings about what is experienced. One might say that all research is about discovery, coming to know truth, and gaining knowledge. Historically, most have viewed science from its empirical perspectives and placed great value on control, prediction, objectivity, and generalizability, terms that will be discussed more thoroughly later. This received perspective has the worldview that a single reality exists and aims to identify truth in objective and replicable ways. Empirical studies are essential for investigating particular variables, but are less helpful in understanding human responses and life experiences.

Whether researchers approach problems from quantitative or qualitative approaches, all are influenced by personal assumptions and beliefs. Some have vigorously argued about the worth of one scientific method over another. The quantitative approach to research has been viewed as successful in measuring and analyzing data, creating studies that can be replicated, and producing results that can be generalized to other populations. The quantitative method is usually referred to as *empirical analytical research*. Some have argued that qualitative methods are less rigorous than quantitative ones. Others say that because qualitative findings are not generalizable, this research method is less trustworthy. Despite the debates, many now agree that qualitative research is an important method for nursing research because some phenomenona or observable events of interest to nursing are less easily measured using quantitative methods. Qualitative methods provide another means for discovering nursing knowledge and have become more respected forms of investigation over the last decade.

Qualitative research is a term often applied to naturalistic investigations, research that involves studying phenomena in places where it is occurring. Qualitative research approaches are based on a perceived perspective or holistic worldview that says there is not a single reality. Instead, reality is viewed as based upon perceptions that differ from person to person and change over time; meaning can only be truly understood if it is associated with a specific situation or context. Qualitative research is about understanding phenomena and finding meaning through examining the pieces that comprise the whole.

51

The most commonly used forms of qualitative nursing research methods are grounded theory, case study, ethnography, and phenomenology. Each method of investigation presents a unique approach to studying the phenomena of interest to nurses and the discipline.

Evidence-based practice has been primarily focused on findings that come from systematic reviews of the literature that use models focused on the effectiveness of interventions. As acceptance has grown for the use of evidence-based practice in nursing, old arguments about the place of qualitative research in this process have arisen. Since research designs such as case, descriptive, and evaluative studies continue to be valued less than empirical ones, it is important to understand the contributions made by qualitative research. Questions of interest to nursing that have not been previously or thoroughly studied are often best investigated using qualitative methods. When new perspectives are introduced to practice, then the use of qualitative investigation may be the best way to gain early understandings that can later be studied using empirical measures. However, reviews of qualitative research about a given topic can also provide meaningful insight into practice issues that can be directly applied in clinical settings.

LEARNING OUTCOMES

On completion of this chapter, the student should be able to do the following:

- Define key concepts in the philosophy of science.
- Identify assumptions underlying the positivist or postpositivist view (positivism) and the constructivist view (constructivism) of research.
- Identify assumptions underlying quantitative (empirical analytical) and the qualitative methods of grounded theory, case study, ethnographic, and phenomenological approaches to research.
- Identify the links between qualitative research and evidence-based practice.

Activity 1

Carper's (1978) seminal work described the four patterns of knowing pertinent to nursing as empirics, moral knowledge, personal knowing, and aesthetic knowing. She described how no single way of knowing provided the entire truth, but each suggests a different perspective of the whole truth. These four patterns of knowing can provide a foundation for truly understanding the diversity and complexity of nursing. Knowledge guides nursing practice! Science is an important way to derive knowledge and is more reliable than instinct or intuition. Research is about asking good questions, questions that generate knowledge. Questions asked by researchers are derived from a variety of different philosophical positions.

1. Before you go any further, and to be sure that you clearly understand the differences between quantitative and qualitative research, take some time to write a clear definition for each of the following terms:

    a.   Quantitative research:

    b.   Qualitative research:

2.   Philosophy is based upon the ways people think about the world. One can find great extremes in worldviews or paradigms. The philosophical perspectives of the researcher influence approaches to research.

    a.   Different philosophers provide windows for considering very different perspectives about the world and allow us to consider how these worldviews can impact the ways research is conducted. Each philosopher you might consider will have a somewhat different perspective about ways to approach research, whether the method is quantitative or qualitative. Go to the *Stanford Encyclopedia of Philosophy* website at http://plato.stanford.edu/ and select "Principal Site: U.S.A." Here you can alphabetically select philosophers to consider. For example, you might want to compare the philosophies of Karl Popper, Edmund Husserel, and Hans-Georg Gadamer. Choose one philosopher and take some time to read about him or her. Then write a 5- to 6-sentence paragraph to describe their main philosophical perspectives. Feel free to use a search engine to find additional websites that provide other information about the selected philosopher.

    b.   Many people view German professor Martin Heidegger (1889-1976) as a leading philosopher relevant to qualitative approaches to research. Many nurses who are qualitative researchers have used his philosophical perspectives while investigating human behaviors applicable to nursing. Go to "Ereignis" at http://www.webcom.com/~paf/ereignis.html and review the many resources about Heidegger. You may also want to look for other websites about Heidegger that provide additional points of view. In 5 to 6 sentences, discuss some of Heidegger's main philosophical perspectives.

Activity 2

In chapter 6 of the textbook, the author provides an overview of qualitative research and introduces a variety of terms that have important implications for understanding qualitative research. Just as it is important to learn the vocabulary associated with quantitative research, this is also true with qualitative research. Take some time to define the following terms and be sure that you can differentiate them:

    a.   Epistemology:

    b.   Ontology:

    c.   Context:

   d. Paradigm:

   e. Constructivism:

   f. Postpositivism:

Activity 3

Review Table 6-1, Basic Beliefs of Research Paradigms, in your textbook and compare the various premises of the constructivist paradigm with those of the postpositivist paradigm. Take some time to consider pain management as an important aspect of cancer care. Given what you already know about clinical care for this problem, suppose you wanted to learn more about relationships between the therapeutics of pain management for people with cancer who were largely cared for by family members. Suppose a case manager, hospice, or home health nurse wanted to facilitate excellence in pain management for this patient. Looking at Table 6-1, how might a researcher view the problem differently if he or she looked at the problem from a constructivist versus a postpositivist paradigm? Take some to time to compare and contrast these two different philosophical positions and identify the differences between these worldviews. Try writing a research question for each paradigm related to this problem.

Activity 4

Chapter 6 describes the philosophical foundations of four qualitative approaches to research: grounded theory, case study, phenomenology, and ethnography. Although other forms of qualitative research exist, these methods are most commonly identified in nursing research.

1. In this activity, you will briefly describe each method, and then state the goal or purpose for each design:

   a. Grounded theory:

   b. Case study:

   c. Phenomenological research:

   d. Ethnographic research:

2. Choose a search engine and investigate each of the four terms online. It may be helpful to combine each of the terms with the word "nursing." Some URLs are suggested for each term, but many others can be found. The goal of this activity is to increase your knowledge about each of the four qualitative research methods, assist you to differentiate among them, and identify ways these research methods are being used by nurses. List three new things you discover for each of the four research methods from your Internet exploration.
   a. Grounded theory:
      Doing it as part of public discourse http://www.habermas.org/grndthry.htm.
      Grounded theory: issues for research in nursing http://www.nursing-standard.co.uk/archives/ns/vol12-52/research.htm.
   b. Case study:
      Using Case Study Methodology in Nursing Research http://www.nova.edu/ssss/QR/QR6-2/zucker.html.
   c. Phenomenology of practice:
      Phenomenology of Practice http://www.phenomenologyonline.com/inquiry/8.html.
      Nursing Informatics http://www.nursing-informatics.com/kwantlen/wwwsites17.html.
   d. Ethnography:
      Ethnography http://en.wikipedia.org/wiki/Ethnography

Activity 5: Web-Based Activity

Unless we have evidence assembled that demonstrates the way we are doing a particular procedure or continuing a specific protocol is less than adequate, most of us assume that because something is being done in nursing practice, it must be correct. Ideas about standards of practice, thoughts about best care, and concerns about quality are causing all practitioners to pay greater attention to questions about the evidence that does or does not support care decisions. While some nurses have embraced the concept of evidence-based care, others continue to be unclear about its implications and how to go about providing this form of care. Because most of the evidence-based studies are focused on quantitative studies often using clinical trials or intervention studies, less is known about the fit between qualitative research and evidence-based care.

Take a few minutes and read the online paper entitled "How can we argue for evidence in nursing?" at http://www.contemporarynurse.com/11.1/11-1p5.htm . This brief article suggests that nurses will make decisions about clinical care based on the best evidence available. However, many questions still exist about behavioral aspects of practice. For example, what is it like to be a young woman with type 1 diabetes who has suffered the complications of blindness and kidney failure, and spends three days a week associating with very ill elderly individuals on dialysis? Think for a few minutes about what that might be like. Then brainstorm to consider what evidence you have about how to best deliver care to this individual if you were the nurse doing hemodialysis. What do you think might be known about care? What might not be known? Although much evidence may exist about the science of the care delivery, what is known that could be considered evidenced-based care in the way nursing care is delivered to meet the holistic needs of this particular client? What kinds of resources and support might be needed that are different from other clients? Qualitative research enables one to investigate questions that are less easily answered through quantitative methods and can provide evidence that can directly impact care delivery.

POST-TEST

1. Identify whether each of the following beliefs reflects the quantitative or the qualitative research method:

    a. _____   Statistical explanation, prediction, and control

    b. _____   Neutral observer

    c. _____   Multiple realities exist

    d. _____   Objectivism valued

    e. _____   Active participant

    f. _____   Experimental

    g. _____   Dialogic

    h. _____   Time and place are important

    i. _____   One reality exists

    j. _____   Values add to understanding the phenomenon

2. Identify whether each of the following indicates an inductive or deductive approach to research:

    a. _____   Researcher uses questionnaires and measurement devices.

    b. _____   Researcher selects participants experienced with the phenomenon of interest.

    c. _____   Researcher primarily uses an analysis process that generates a numerical summary.

    d. _____   Researcher uses an intensive approach of self in data collection.

    e. _____   Researcher primarily uses a narrative summary for conclusions of analysis.

3. Identify which of the following descriptions fits each form of qualitative research:

    A = Grounded theory
    B = Phenomenology
    C = Case study
    D = Ethnography

    a. _____   Designed to inductively develop a theory based on observations.

b. _____ Describes patterns of behavior of people within a culture.

c. _____ Culture is a fundamental value underlying this form of research.

d. _____ This form of research answers questions about meaning.

e. _____ This form of research can assist us in understanding differences and similarities.

Please check with your instructor for the answers to the post-test.

REFERENCES

Carper B (1978). Fundamental patterns of knowing in nursing. *Adv Nurs Sci* 1(1), 13–23.

Ereignis. Accessed July 21, 2005 from http://www.webcom.com/~paf/ereignis.html.

Kaminiski J (2002). Nursing Informatics. Accessed June 22, 2005 from http://www.nursing-informatics.com/kwantlen/wwwsites17.html.

Sheldon L (1998). Grounded Theory: Issues for Research in Nursing. Accessed June 22, 2005 from http://www.nursing-standard.co.uk/archives/ns/vol12-52/research.htm.

Stanford Encyclopedia of Philosophy. Accessed July 21, 2005 from http://plato.stanford.edu/.

Street A (2001). How can we argue for evidence in nursing? *Contemp Nurs* 11(1):5–8. Accessed July 21, 2005 from http://www.contemporarynurse.com/11.1/11-1p5.htm.

van Manen M (2000). Phenomenology of Practice. Accessed June 22, 2005 from http://www.phenomenologyonline.com/inquiry/8.html.

Zucker D (2001). Using Case Study Methodology in Nursing Research. Accessed June 22, 2005 from http://www.nova.edu/ssss/QR/QR6-2/zucker.html.

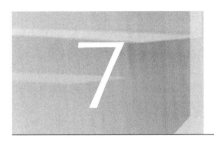

7 Qualitative Approaches to Research

INTRODUCTION

Qualitative research continues to gain recognition as a sound method for investigating the complex human phenomena less easily explored using quantitative methods. Qualitative research methods provide ways to address both the science and art of nursing. Qualitative methods are especially well-suited to address phenomena related to health and illness that are of interest to nurses and nursing practice. Nurse researchers and investigators from other disciplines are continuing to discover the increased value of findings obtained through qualitative studies. Nurses can be better prepared to critique the appropriateness of a research design and identify the usefulness of the study findings when the unique differences between quantitative and qualitative research approaches are understood.

Although many designs of qualitative research might be considered, five methods are most commonly used by nurses. These methods are phenomenology, grounded theory, historical research, ethnography, and case study. A newer methodology known as community-based participatory research that is gaining increased respect by nursing scientists who are investigating behavioral phenomena is also described in this chapter. Understanding and care are concepts related to behaviors that are important to nurses in the practice of clinical nursing care in a variety of settings across the lifespan. Each of these qualitative methods allows the researcher to approach the phenomena of interest from a different perspective. Each offers the investigator a different perspective and suggests findings that address different realms of human experience.

LEARNING OUTCOMES

On completion of this chapter, the student should be able to do the following:

- Identify connections among worldview, research question, and research method.
- Recognize the use of qualitative research for nursing.
- Identify the processes of phenomenological, grounded theory, ethnographic, and case study methods.
- Recognize appropriate use of historical methods.

- Recognize appropriate use of community-based participatory research methods.
- Discuss significant issues that arise in conducting qualitative research in relation to such topics as ethics, criteria for judging scientific rigor, combination of research methods, and use of computers to assist data management.
- Discuss qualitative research as a source of evidence for clinical decision-making.
- Apply the critiquing criteria to evaluate a report of qualitative research.

Activity 1

The reasons for selecting a qualitative design rather than a quantitative one are based upon the type of research question asked and the study purpose. Recognizing the different characteristics of qualitative research from those of quantitative research enables the nurse to better understand the way the study was conducted, and interpret the research report findings. Clear understandings about qualitative research can also assist the nurse to better understand applications for the findings from these studies.

1. Complete the following statements related to qualitative research characteristics.

   a. Qualitative research combines the _____ and _____ natures of nursing to better understand the human experience.

   b. Qualitative research is used to study human experience and life context in

      _____ _____.

   c. Life context is the matrix of human-human-environment relationships that emerge over the course of _____ _____.

   d. Qualitative researchers study the _____ _____ of individuals as they carry on their usual activities of daily living, which might occur at home, work, or school.

   e. The number of participants or subjects in a qualitative study is usually _____ than the number in a quantitative study.

   f. Qualitative studies are intended to explore _____ _____ or _____ _____ in order to better understand the meanings ascribed by individuals living the experience.

   g. The choice to use either quantitative or qualitative methods is guided by the

      _____ _____.

   h. One research method is not better than another; it has to do with the _____ between one's worldview, the research question, and the research method.

2. Match the following terms with the appropriate definitions:

A. Theoretical sampling
B. Emic
C. Etic
D. Data saturation
E. Secondary sources
F. Bracketed
G. Case study method
H. Grounded theory method
I. Domains
J. Key informants

a. _____ Information becomes repetitive

b. _____ Select experiences to help the researcher test ideas and gather complete information about developing concepts

c. _____ Outsider's view

d. _____ Identify personal biases about the phenomenon

e. _____ Insider's view

f. _____ Symbolic categories

g. _____ Individuals willing to teach investigator about the phenomenon

h. _____ In-depth description of the phenomenon

i. _____ Provide another perspective of the phenomenon

j. _____ Inductive approach to develop theory about social processes

3. Six qualitative research methods are discussed in the textbook in relation to five basic research elements. Use your textbook to compare research elements of each of the different types of qualitative methods. Briefly describe a key aspect of each element for the different qualitative methods. This activity will assist you to compare and contrast the similarities and differences in these methods.
   a. Element 1: Identifying the phenomenon
      1. Phenomenology

      2. Grounded theory method

      3. Ethnography

      4. Historical research

      5. Case study

      6. Community-based participatory research

b.   Element 2: Structuring the study
  1.   Phenomenology

  2.   Grounded theory method

  3.   Ethnography

  4.   Historical research

  5.   Case study

  6.   Community-based participatory research

c.   Element 3: Gathering the data
  1.   Phenomenology

  2.   Grounded theory method

  3.   Ethnography

  4.   Historical research

  5.   Case study

  6.   Community-based participatory research

d.   Element 4: Analyzing the data
  1.   Phenomenology

  2.   Grounded theory method

  3.   Ethnography

  4.   Historical research

  5.   Case study

  6.   Community-based participatory research

e.   Element 5: Describing the findings
  1.   Phenomenology

  2.   Grounded theory method

  3.   Ethnography

4. Historical research

5. Case study

6. Community-based participatory research

4. Take some time to think about an area of clinical practice that is of special interest to you. Consider questions or practice issues related to the clinical area. What kinds of problems do you think might be researched using qualitative perspectives? Make a list of two or three topics or problems that could be researched. Now identify the one that is of most interest to you. Based upon the work you have just completed above about the five elements of research methods, give some critical thought about the type of qualitative research that would be most appropriate for studying the identified problem. Once you have selected the type of qualitative research you would use, be prepared to explain the reasons for your choice.

Activity 2

The literature review usually provides the background and significance for understanding a research problem. All qualitative research methods do not include literature reviews, or if they do, they may tend to be much briefer than ones found in quantitative studies. The study in your text (Appendix C) entitled "Social Role Experiences of Women Living with Rheumatoid Arthritis" by Plach, Stevens, and Moss (2004) has included a brief discussion about Americans diagnosed with rheumatoid arthritis. Read the literature review at the beginning of this study report carefully, and then answer the following questions:

1. What is the main theme of the literature review?

2. How does this literature review introduce the reader to important problems associated with rheumatoid arthritis that might require research? What are the key points that the authors identify about the disease?

3. The authors say that this qualitative study followed a quantitative one. What was it in the earlier study that made a follow-up qualitative method an appropriate means to continue research in this area?

Activity 3

Read the methods section of the Plach, Stevens, and Moss (2004) report in Appendix C of your text and answer the following questions:

1. What research design was used to conduct this research study?

2. Describe the sample in this study.

3. What important procedures and methods were used to collect data in this study?

4. What methods were used during data analysis?

Activity 4

Qualitative research has many uses for nursing practice. After reading the Plach, Stevens, and Moss (2004) report in Appendix C of your text and considering the study findings, list some things learned and consider ways this research might be applicable to nursing practice.

Activity 5

Five qualitative methods of research are the phenomenological, grounded theory, ethnographic, case study, and historical methods. For each characteristic listed below, indicate which method of qualitative research it describes. Use the abbreviations from the key provided.

  Key:
  A = Phenomenological
  B = Grounded theory
  C = Ethnographic
  D = Historical
  E = Case study

  a. _____   Uses primary and secondary sources

  b. _____   Uses "emic" and "etic" views of subjects' worlds

  c. _____   Research questions are action- or change-oriented

  d. _____   Central meanings arise from subjects' descriptions of lived experience

  e. _____   Truth is a lived experience

f. _____ Uses theoretical sampling to analyze data

g. _____ Studies the peculiarities and commonalities of a specific case

h. _____ Discovers "domains" to analyze data

i. _____ Provides insight on the past and serves as a guide to the present and future

j. _____ Establishes fact, probability, or possibility

k. _____ States individuals' history is a dimension of the present

l. _____ Attempts to discover underlying social forces that shape human behavior

m. _____ Seldom found in nursing journals

n. _____ Interviews "key informants"

o. _____ Presents data as a synthesized chronicle

p. _____ Focuses on describing cultural groups

q. _____ Establishes reliability through external and internal criticism

r. _____ Researcher "brackets" personal bias or perspective

s. _____ Can include quantitative and/or qualitative data

t. _____ Subjects are currently experiencing a circumstance

u. _____ Collects remembered information from subjects

v. _____ Involves "field work"

w. _____ Describes events from the past

x. _____ May use photographs to describe current behavioral practices

y. _____ Uses symbolic interaction as a theoretical base

z. _____ Uses an inductive approach to understanding basic social processes

Activity 6

Critical thinking is an important aspect of all research. It is important to take some time and carefully consider all aspects of the research process prior to beginning. Based on the five methods of qualitative research described in the textbook, answer the following questions:

a. Select a qualitative method you found especially interesting and explain the two things you find appealing about this method.

   b. Identify three subject areas for which this method might be helpful in developing nursing knowledge:

     (1)

     (2)

     (3)

   c. Choose one of these subject areas and identify a research question to be studied.

   d. Describe the data-collection methods you would use for this study.

   e. Identify the characteristics of the study subjects, where you will locate them, how many subjects you might include, and why.

   f. Briefly explain an important aspect of data analysis using this qualitative method.

   g. Describe how you might use the knowledge gained from this study in nursing practice.

Activity 7: Web-Based Activity

Qualitative research is a way to develop knowledge about the complexity of the human health experience that occurs within a contextual setting during everyday life and over the lifespan. Chapter 7 in your textbook suggests that the use of qualitative research methods can provide evidence as findings are generated to (a) guide nursing practice, (b) contribute to development of instruments that can be used in quantitative research studies, and (c) develop nursing theory that can guide practice.

    Go to *The Qualitative Report* http://www.nova.edu/ssss/QR/web.html and see the large number of sources that can provide you additional understanding about qualitative research and assist you to understand better how the evidence produced by qualitative research is directly linked to nursing education, clinical practice, and research. Take some time to look over a few of these sites. You may want to select one that is related to the form of qualitative research that you have found especially intriguing. It is important that you begin to have some sense of the plentifulness of work that is being done by nurses and others using qualitative methods. Although some continue to question the usefulness of these methods, the respect and use of these means of scientific inquiry are continuing to grow and be more greatly respected.

After you have finished looking around, scroll down and select "Action Research on the Web." When the new page opens, click on "Research" and then choose "Action Research electronic Reports (AReR)." Select "Cultural attitudes / beliefs about pain: A collaborative inquiry journey." Read through this article and then answer the following questions:

a. What is collaborative inquiry?

b. How is research conducted using this method?

c. Review Table 1 "Questions on cultural attitudes towards pain" and Table 2 "The experience of pain: how do we express pain?" After you review these findings, discuss how this might become evidence for education or clinical practice.

POST-TEST

For questions 1 through 5, answer True (T) or False (F).

1. _____ Qualitative research focuses on the whole of human experience in naturalistic settings.

2. _____ External criticism in historical research refers to the authenticity of data sources.

3. _____ In qualitative research one would expect the number of subjects participating to be as large as those usually found in quantitative studies.

4. _____ The researcher is viewed as the major instrument for data collection.

5. _____ Qualitative studies strive to eliminate extraneous variables.

6. To what does the term "saturation" in qualitative research refer?
   a. Data repetition
   b. Subject exhaustion
   c. Researcher exhaustion
   d. Sample size

7. Data, in qualitative research, are often collected by which of the following procedures?
   a. Questionnaires sent out to subjects
   b. Observation of subjects in naturalistic settings
   c. Interviews
   d. All are correct

8. The qualitative method that uses symbolic interaction as the theoretical base for research is known as which of the following?
   a. Phenomenology
   b. Grounded theory
   c. Ethnography
   d. Historical method

9. What is the qualitative method that attempts to construct the meaning of the lived experience of human phenomena?
   a. Phenomenology
   b. Grounded theory
   c. Ethnography
   d. Historical method
   e. Case study
   f. Community-based participatory research

10. What is the qualitative research method most appropriate for answering the question "What changes in nursing practice occurred after the Vietnam War?"
    a. Phenomenology
    b. Grounded theory
    c. Ethnography
    d. Historical method
    e. Case study
    f. Community-based participatory research

11. What qualitative research method would be most appropriate for studying the impact of culture on the health behaviors of urban Hispanic youth?
    a. Phenomenology
    b. Grounded theory
    c. Ethnography
    d. Historical method
    e. Case study
    f. Community-based participatory research

12. What qualitative method would be most appropriate for studying a family's experience with cystic fibrosis?
    a. Phenomenology
    b. Grounded theory
    c. Ethnography
    d. Historical method
    e. Case study
    f. Community-based participatory research

13. What qualitative method would you use to study the spread of HIV/AIDS in an urban area?
    a. Phenomenology
    b. Grounded theory
    c. Ethnography
    d. Historical method
    e. Case study
    f. Community-based participatory research

14. Which data analysis process is not used with grounded theory methodology?
    a. Bracketing
    b. Axial coding
    c. Theoretical sampling
    d. Open coding

Please check with your instructor for the answers to the post-test.

REFERENCES

Denham SA (1999). Family health in an economically disadvantaged population, *J Fam Nurs* 5(2):184–213.

Lovering S (2004). Cultural attitudes / beliefs about pain: A collaborative inquiry journey. Action Research electronic Reports. Retrieved July 21, 2005 from http://www2.fhs.usyd.edu.au/arow/arer/022.htm.

Plach SK, Stevens PE, Moss VA (2004). Social role experiences of women living with rheumatoid arthritis, *J Fam Nurs* 10(1):33–49.

Evaluating Qualitative Research

INTRODUCTION

Qualitative research provides an opportunity to generate new knowledge about phenomena less easily studied with empirical or quantitative methods. Nurse researchers are increasingly using qualitative methods to explore holistic aspects less easily investigated with objective measures. In qualitative research, the data are less likely to involve numbers and most likely will include text derived from interviews, focus groups, observation, field notes, or other methods. The data tend to be mostly narrative or written words that require content rather than statistical analysis. The important contributions being made to nursing knowledge through qualitative studies make it important for nurses to possess skills that enable them to evaluate and critique qualitative research reports.

This chapter describes the criteria needed to evaluate and critique qualitative research reports. Qualitative researchers should provide the insider or emic view of the phenomenon being studied. Qualitative investigators often use a more conversational tone than what is found in quantitative research, and use quotations as a way to present the findings. Page limits in journals greatly constrain the ways investigators can present the richness of the data. Quotations selected must be chosen as exemplars that make the themes understandable to the reader. Published research reports, whether they are quantitative or qualitative, must be viewed by the reviewers as having scientific merit, demonstrate rigor in the research conducted, present new knowledge, and be of interest to the journal's readers. Qualitative research should offer evidence to enhance understanding or increase knowledge about a specific phenomenon; it may also have strong implications for the way nursing practice is conceptualized and delivered.

LEARNING OUTCOMES

On completion of this chapter, the student should be able to do the following:

- Identify the influence of stylistic considerations on the presentation of a qualitative research report.
- Identify the criteria for critiquing a qualitative research report.

- Evaluate the strengths and weaknesses of a qualitative research report.
- Describe the applicability of the findings of a qualitative research report.
- Construct a critique of a qualitative research report.

Activity 1

The methods of presentation in qualitative research reports are different than those in quantitative studies. Nurses doing qualitative research reports are challenged to present the richness of the data within the restrictions of publication guidelines.

Review the article entitled "Social Role Experiences of Women Living with Rheumatoid Arthritis" by Plach, Stevens, and Moss (2004) (Appendix C in the text) to identify the ways the researchers stylistically presented the rich data. In the finding section entitled "No Roles Left Untouched by RA," the researchers describe several aspects of this experience and give examples from the data to describe what is implied. Carefully read this section and identify the descriptive examples or quotations that summarize the key points.

Activity 2

The findings of qualitative studies describe or explain a phenomenon within a specific context. The findings are not usually intended to be generalizable to other groups, which means that people who want to apply the findings to others have the responsibility to validate whether the findings are applicable in a different setting and with other people or populations.

The article by Plach, Stevens, and Moss (2004) (Appendix C in the text) describes the experience of a number of women who are living with rheumatoid arthritis. The discussion section compares this study's findings with other things in the current literature.

1. What does the study conclude about rheumatoid arthritis as a chronic illness?

2. What does the study say about the impact that developmental changes have upon social roles?

3. What do the authors suggest about the implications of feminist ideas and women's roles?

4. What do the authors of this study tell us about support networks?

5. What do the authors suggest about generalizing the findings?

Activity 3

Critiquing qualitative research enables the nurse to make sense out of the research report, build on the body of knowledge about human phenomena, and consider how knowledge might be applicable to nursing. Learning and applying a critiquing process is the first step in this process.

1. Review Box 8-1 in the text and match the qualitative research process in Column A with the activity in Column B. Some steps are used more than once.

Column A
A. Subject selection
B. Study method
C. Researcher perspective
D. Data analysis
E. Application of findings
F. Findings description
G. Study design

Column B

a. _____ The purpose of the study is clearly stated.

b. _____ Audiotaped interviews were used to collect phenomeno-logical data.

c. _____ Do the participants recognize the experience as their own?

d. _____ Purposive sampling was used.

e. _____ Data are clearly reported in the research report.

f. _____ The researcher has remained true to the findings.

g. _____ Recommendations for future research are made.

h. _____ The phenomenon of interest is clearly identified.

i. _____ Participant observation was done in an ethnography.

2. Define the following terms:
   a. Credibility:

   b. Auditability:

   c. Fittingness:

   d. Saturation:

   e. Trustworthiness:

Activity 4: Web-Based Activity

The Internet can be a valuable tool in gaining insight into qualitative research topics. Searching the term *qualitative research* can be a way to gain additional understanding about many aspects of this research approach. However, it is essential to identify a few quality starting points for your investigation. The Association for Information Systems has a page entitled "Qualitative Research in Information Systems" http://www.qual.auckland.ac.nz/ on the conduct, evaluation, and publication of qualitative research. You will find some valuable information about qualitative studies at this site. The University of Alberta's "International Institute for Qualitative Methodology" http://www.ualberta.ca/~iiqm/ is an excellent place to locate information about conferences, journals, training, and international research. Another good site is Judy Norris's "QualPage" http://www.qualitativeresearch.uga.edu/QualPage/, a valuable resource for learning more about the various methods of qualitative research.

The Cochrane Collaboration http://www.cochrane.org/index0.htm is an international nonprofit organization whose purpose is to produce and disseminate reviews of health care interventions and clinical trials that provide evidence for practice.

You may want to spend some time reviewing these websites to learn more about the state of qualitative research methods. Your instructor may want to assign some particular activities from these websites to assist you in learning about qualitative research.

Activity 5: Evidence-Based Practice Activity

Evidence-based care using qualitative research is a scientific area still being developed, but certainly one that is vitally important in answering many of the questions of interest to nursing. While most now recognize the value that qualitative methods provide in answering scientific questions, some questions about rigor still exist. In chapter 7 of your text, you will find a discussion of triangulation. *Triangulation* refers to comparison of findings derived from two or more data gathering procedures or sources of information. This technique enables one to assess emerging findings for the extent of consistency or inconsistency among data derived from different sources. For example, the article entitled "Social Role Experiences of Women Living with Rheumatoid Arthritis" by Plach, Stevens, and Moss (2004) (Appendix C of your text) describes the qualitative arm of a triangulated study. Look at the reference pages of this article and note that Dr. Plach has cited a number of other articles about her research in this area. You may want to obtain a copy of the Plach, Heidrich, and Waite (2003) article that describes the quantitative aspects of this triangulated study.

a. What was the quantitative arm of this larger study about?

b. What was the conclusion reached in the quantitative study?

c. Did the triangulated study (in other words, the qualitative portion of the study) support the quantitative research findings?

d. Did the qualitative findings seem to add anything to the quantitative findings?

POST-TEST

For questions 1 through 6, answer True (T) or False (F).

1. _____ Qualitative research findings are generalizable to other groups.

2. _____ Findings from qualitative research designs are viewed as less credible by nurse researchers than those gained from quantitative studies.

3. _____ Auditability is an important aspect of evaluating a qualitative research report.

4. _____ The style of a qualitative research report differs from that of a quantitative research report.

5. _____ Some journal publication guidelines may impede the qualitative researcher's ability to convey the richness of the data.

6. _____ Journal reviewer's guidelines usually allow for the extra pages that qualitative researchers might need to provide the detail of their rich data.

7. _____ means that others should be able to identify the thinking, decisions, and methods used by the researcher(s) when they conducted the research study.

8. _____ means that the study findings fit well outside the study situation.

9. _____ means that the research informants can identify the reported findings as their own experience.

10. _____ is the term usually applied to qualitative research to judge the validity and reliability of qualitative data.

Please check with your instructor for the answers to the post-test.

REFERENCES

The Cochrane Collaboration. Accessed July 21, 2005 from http://www.cochrane.org/index0.htm.

Myers MD. "Qualitative Research in Information Systems," *MIS Quarterly* (21:2), June 1997, pp. 241-242. *MISQ Discovery*, archival version, June 1997, http://www.misq.org/discovery/MISQD_isworld/. *MISQ Discovery*, updated version, last modified www.qual.auckland.ac.nz. Retrieved June 22, 2005.

Norris J: QualPage: Resources for Qualitative Research. Retrieved June 22, 2005 from http://www.qualitativeresearch.uga.edu/QualPage/.

Plach SK, Stevens PE, Moss VA (2004) Social role experiences of women living with rheumatoid arthritis, *J Family Nurs* 10(1):33-49.

Plach SK, Heidrich SM, Waite RM (2003). Relationship of social role quality to psychological well-being in women with rheumatoid arthritis, *Res Nurs Health* 26(3):190-202.

University of Alberta: International Institute for Qualitative Methodology. Accessed July 21, 2005 from http://www.ualberta.ca/~iiqm/.

Introduction to Quantitative Research

INTRODUCTION

The term *research design* is used to describe the overall plan of a particular study. The design is the researcher's plan for answering specific research questions in the most accurate and efficient way possible. In quantitative research, the plan outlines how the hypotheses will be tested. The design ties together the present research problem, the knowledge of the past, and the implications for the future. Thus the choice of a design reflects the researcher's experience, expertise, knowledge, and biases.

LEARNING OUTCOMES

On completion of this chapter, the student should be able to do the following:

- Define research design.
- Identify the purpose of research design.
- Define control as it affects research design.
- Compare and contrast the elements that affect control.
- Begin to evaluate what degree of control should be exercised in research design.
- Define internal validity.
- Identify the threats to internal validity.
- Define external validity.
- Identify the conditions that affect external validity.
- Identify the links between the study design and evidence-based practice.
- Evaluate research design using critiquing questions.

Activity 1

Match the definition of the terms in Column A with the research design terms in Column B. Each term is used no more than once, and not all terms will be used. Check the glossary for help with terms.

Column A

1. _____ A sample of subjects similar to one another

2. _____ The subject's responses to being studied

3. _____ Methods to keep the study conditions constant during the study

4. _____ Consideration whether the study is possible and practical to conduct

5. _____ The vehicle for hypothesis testing or answering research questions

6. _____ Process to ensure every subject has an equal chance of being selected

7. _____ Degree to which a research study is consistent within itself

8. _____ Degree to which the study results can be applied to the larger population

9. _____ All parts of a study follow logically from the problem statement

Column B

a. External validity
b. Internal validity
c. Accuracy
d. Research design
e. Control
f. Random sampling
g. Feasibility
h. Homogenous sampling
i. Objectivity
j. Reactivity

Activity 2

For each of the following situations, identify the type of threat to internal validity from the list below. Then explain the reason this is a problem, and suggest how this problem can be corrected.

History	Mortality
Instrumentation	Selection bias
Maturation	Testing

1. The researcher tested the effectiveness of a new method of teaching drug dosage and solution calculations to nursing students using a standardized calculation exam at the beginning, midpoint, and end of a 2-week course.

2. In a study of the results of a hypertension teaching program conducted at a senior center, the blood pressures taken by volunteers using their personal equipment were compared before and after the program.

3. A major increase in cigarette taxes occurs during a one-year follow-up study of the impact of a smoking cessation program.

4. The smoking cessation rates of an experimental group consisting of volunteers for a smoking cessation program were compared with the results of a control group of people who wanted to quit on their own without a special program.

5. Thirty percent of the subjects dropped out of an experimental study of the effect of a job-training program on employment for homeless women. Over 90% of the dropouts were single homeless women with at least two preschool children, while the majority of subjects successfully completing the program had no preschool children.

6. Nurses on a maternity unit want to study the effect of a new hospital-based teaching program on mothers' confidence in caring for their newborn infants. The researchers mail out a survey one month after discharge.

Activity 3

The term *research design* is an all-encompassing term for the overall plan to answer the research questions, including the method and specific plans to control other factors that could influence the results of the study. To become acquainted with the major elements in the design of a study, read the Koniak-Griffin et al. (2003) article (Appendix A in the text) and answer the following questions:

a. What was the setting for the study?

b. Who were the subjects?

c. How was the sample selected?

d. What information was missing?

e. Was this a homogenous sample?

f. How were variables measured and constancy maintained?

g. Which group served as the control group?

Activity 4

Use the critiquing criteria in chapter 9 to critique the research design of the Koniak-Griffin et al. (2003) study (Appendix A in the text). Explain your answers.

1. Is the design appropriate?

2. Is the control consistent with the research design?

3. Think about the feasibility of this study. Is this a study that would be expected of a master's student in nursing? Of a doctoral student? Explain the reasoning behind your answer.

4. Does the design logically flow from problem, framework, literature review, and hypothesis?

5. What are the threats to internal validity and how did the investigators control for each?

6. What are the threats to external validity and how did the investigators control for each?

Activity 5: Web-Based Activity

Assume you are thinking about submitting a proposal to National Institute of Nursing Research (NINR). You are a multi-talented researcher and are equally qualified to conduct either qualitative or quantitative research. You are curious about the number of grants awarded that would be considered quantitative or qualitative. Start at the NINR website and describe how you could use this site to get a sense of the qualitative/quantitative ratio.

Go to http://ninr.nih.gov/ninr/. Click on each of the following in order:

Research Funding and Programs
Division of Extramural Activities
All Funded Research Awards
FY 2002 or FY 2003

Review the studies that appear. Do these titles give you enough information to determine if the awarded grant was qualitative or quantitative in nature? Read through the first 10 citations and label them as either qualitative or quantitative.

Note: URLs for websites may change. If you receive an error message at the URL listed above, go to your favorite search engine and type in, "national institute for nursing research;" this should lead you to the desired site.

An excellent source of information about both quantitative and qualitative studies can be your own university library. Go to your campus home page and type in "library," then type in "research" or "nursing research." This can be an excellent source for full-text journals; however, they are usually password-protected, so you will need to obtain a password from your library to access them.

Activity 6: Evidence-Based Practice Activity

Review Table 2-3 "Levels of Evidence: Rating System for the Hierarchy of Evidence" from your text below. For each level of evidence, indicate whether the evidence is (A) expert opinion, (B) qualitative, (C) quantitative, (D) combination of qualitative and quantitative, or (E) anecdotal.

Table 2-3   Levels of Evidence: Rating System for the Hierarchy of Evidence

Assessing Level of Evidence	Source of Evidence
Level I	Evidence from a systematic review or meta-analysis of all relevant randomized controlled trials (RCTs) or evidence-based clinical practice guidelines based on systematic reviews of RCTs
Level II	Evidence obtained from at least one well-designed RCT
Level III	Evidence obtained from well-designed controlled trials without randomization (e.g., quasiexperimental study)
Level IV	Evidence from nonexperimental studies (e.g., case-control and cohort studies)
Level V	Evidence from systematic reviews of descriptive and qualitative studies
Level VI	Evidence from a single descriptive or qualitative study
Level VII	Evidence from the opinion of authorities and/or reports of expert committees

(Modified from Melnyk and Fineout-Overholt, 2005.)

1. Level I:

2. Level II:

3. Level III:

4. Level IV:

5. Level V:

7. Level VI:

POST-TEST

1. Review the Davison et al. (2003) study "Provision of individualized information to men and their partners to facilitate treatment decision making in prostate cancer" (Appendix D of the text). Briefly assess the major components of the research design.

    a. Use your own words to state the purpose of the study.

    b. What is the setting for the study?

    c. Who are the subjects?

    d. How is the sample selected?

    e. What is the research treatment?

    f. How do the researchers attempt to control elements affecting the results of the study?

2. Fill in the blanks by selecting from the following list of terms. Not all terms will be used.

Constancy	Mortality
Control	Internal validity
Feasibility	External validity
Selection bias	Accuracy
Reliability	History
Maturation	

    a. _____ is used to hold steady the conditions of the study.

    b. _____ is used to describe that all aspects of a study logically follow from the problem statement.

    c. The believability between this study and the world at large is known as _____.

    d. The developmental, biological, or psychological processes known as _____ operate within a person over time and may influence the results of a study.

    e. Time, subject availability, equipment, money, experience, and ethics are factors influencing the _____ of a study.

    f. Selection bias, mortality, maturation, instrumentation, testing, and history influence the _____ of a study.

    g. Voluntary (rather than random) assignment to an experimental or control condition creates a situation known as _____.

Please check with your instructor for the answers to the post-test.

REFERENCES

Davison BJ, Goldenberg SL, Gleave ME, et al. (2003). Provision of individualized information to men and their partners to facilitate treatment decision making in prostate cancer, *Oncol Nurs Forum* 30(1):107-114.

Koniak-Griffin D, Verzemnieks IL, Anderson NLR, et al. (2003). Nurse visitation for adolescent mothers: Two-year infant health and maternal outcomes, *Nurs Res* 52(2):127-136.

National Institute of Nursing Research. Retrieved July 21, 2005 from http://ninr.nih.gov/ninr/.

10 Experimental and Quasiexperimental Designs

INTRODUCTION

This chapter contains exercises for two categories of design: experimental and quasiexperimental. These types of designs allow researchers to test the effects of nursing actions and make statements about cause-and-effect relationships. Therefore, they can be very helpful in testing solutions to nursing practice problems. However, a researcher chooses the design that allows a given situation or problem to be studied in the most accurate and effective way possible. Thus, not all problems are amenable to immediate study by these two types of designs. Rather, the choice of design is dependent on the development of knowledge relevant to the problem, plus the researcher's knowledge, experience, expertise, preferences, and resources.

LEARNING OUTCOMES

On completion of this chapter, the student should be able to do the following:

- Identify the components of experimental and quasiexperimental research designs.
- Compare and contrast experimental and quasiexperimental research designs.
- Critique the type of design used in experimental, quasiexperimental, and program evaluation studies.
- Critique the application potential of the findings of specific experimental and quasiexperimental studies.

Activity 1

Fill in the blank for each of the following descriptions with a term selected from the list of types of experimental and quasiexperimental designs. Each term is used only once and not all terms may be used. Consult the glossary for assistance with definition of terms.

  After-only experiment
  After-only nonequivalent control group
  Experimental
  Evaluation research
  Nonequivalent control group
  Solomon four-group
  Time series

1. _____ designs are particularly suitable for testing cause-and-effect relationships because they help eliminate potential alternative explanations (threats to validity) for the findings.

2. The type of design that has two groups identical to the true experimental design plus an experimental after-group and a control after-group is known as a(n) _____ design.

3. A research approach used when only one group is available to study for trends over a longer period of time is called a(n) _____ design.

4. The _____ design is also known as the post-test–only control group design in which neither the experimental group nor the control group is pretested.

5. If a researcher wants to compare results obtained from an experimental group with a control group, but was unable to conduct pretests or to randomly assign subjects to groups, the study would be known as a(n) _____ design.

6. The _____ design includes three properties: randomization, control, and manipulation.

7. When subjects are unable to be randomly assigned into experimental and control groups but are able to be pretested and post-tested, the design is known as a(n) _____ design.

Activity 2

Review the study by Koniak-Griffin et al. (2003) "Nurse visitation for adolescent mothers: Two-year infant health and maternal outcomes" found in Appendix A of the text, and then answer the following questions.

1. What is the name of the design used in this study?

2. Would this design be classified as experimental or quasiexperimental? Explain.

3. What are the events which could be labeled antecedent variables and intervening variables in the study that could have affected internal validity?

    a. Which events would be labeled an antecedent variable?

    b. Which would be labeled an intervening variable?

4. List the implications of this study for nursing practice.

Activity 3

The education department in a large hospital wants to test a program to educate and change nurse's attitudes regarding pain management. They have a questionnaire that measures nurses' knowledge and attitudes about pain. Your responsibility is to design a study to examine the outcome of this intervention program.

1. You decide to use a Solomon four-group design. Complete the chart below with an X to indicate which of the four groups receive the pretest and post-test pain questionnaire, and which receive the experimental teaching program.

	Pretest	Teaching	Post-Test
Group A	_____	_____	_____
Group B	_____	_____	_____
Group C	_____	_____	_____
Group D	_____	_____	_____

2. How would you assign nurses to each of the four groups?

3. What would you use as a pretest for the groups receiving the pretest?

4. What is the experimental treatment?

5. What is the outcome measure for each group?

6. Based on your reading, for what types of issues is this design particularly effective?

7.   What is the major advantage for this type of design?

8.   What is a disadvantage for this type of design?

Activity 4

For each of the following descriptions of experimental or quasiexperimental studies, identify the type of design used in the study and the advantages and disadvantages of this design.

1.   The purpose of this study was to evaluate the effect of the Foster Pain Intervention (FPI) on pain and mobility. Seventy women who were scheduled for a hysterectomy completed the Preoperative Self-Efficacy Scale. The first 35 women who met the criteria were assigned to the control group, and the next 35 were assigned to the intervention group. Both groups received routine preoperative information. Those in the intervention group also received the Foster Pain Intervention information. On the first and second postoperative days the Patient Mobility and the Observer Mobility Scales were scored (Heye et al. 2002).

    a.   What type of design was used?

    b.   What are the advantages of this design?

    c.   What are the disadvantages of this design?

2.   The purpose of this study was to determine the effectiveness of a thermal mattress in stabilizing and maintaining body temperature during the transport of newborns who weigh less than 1500 g. Three rectal temperature measurements of two groups of neonates were compared. Between April 1998 and October 1999 the treatment group of 100 infants was placed on a thermal mattress during transport from a referring hospital to the tertiary care center. Comparable rectal temperatures of 91 infants transported between April 1995 and March 1996 without a thermal mattress were obtained from medical records (L'Herault et al. 2001).

    a.   What type of design was used? (Think it through; this design is a combination of two of the designs addressed in the text.)

    b.   Now really put your thinking cap on and see if you can think of why this would be a reasonable choice of design. (Hint: An ethical principle and standards of care are involved.)

3.   The purpose of the study was to evaluate the effectiveness of interventions provided by a Community Mental Health Team in reducing stress in caregivers of individuals with dementia. Following initial multidisciplinary assessment, all caregivers of individuals with dementia were invited to participate; 26 caregivers consented and participated in all stages

of data collection. Data were collected at initial assessment, and again at 3 and 6 months using the Caregiver Strain Index (Hoskins et al. 2005).

    a.   What type of design was used?

    b.   What are the advantages of this design?

    c.   What are the disadvantages of this design?

Activity 5

1.   You may be questioning why anyone would use a quasiexperimental design if an experimental design has the advantage of being so much stronger in detecting cause-and-effect relationships and enabling the researcher to generalize the results to a wider population. In what instances might it be advantageous to use a quasiexperimental design?

2.   What must the researcher do in order to generalize the findings from a quasiexperimental research study?

3.   What must a clinician do before application of research findings into practice?

Activity 6: Web-Based Activity

In this activity, you are looking for experimental nursing research studies.

1.   Go to www.PubMed.gov and type in "experimental studies nursing." Look at the top of the list of items. How many articles were found?

2.   Find the article by Barkauskas, Lusk, and Eakin (2005) "Selecting control interventions for clinical outcome studies." Is this an actual experimental study? If not, what is it?

3.   Now click on the "Limits" tab near the top. In the "Publication Types" drop-down menu, choose the option "Randomized Control Trial." Click on "Go." How many articles were found with this limit set?

4.   Go to the article by White-Traut et al. (2005) "Feeding readiness in preterm infants: The relationship between preterm behavioral state and feeding readiness behaviors and efficiency during transition from gavage to oral feeding." Is this an actual experimental study? If not, what type of study is it?

☀ Activity 7: Evidence-Based Practice Activity

When using evidence-based practice strategies, the first step is to decide which level of evidence a research article provides. Review Table 2-3, Levels of Evidence: Rating System for the Hierarchy of Evidence below from your textbook.

Table 2-3   Levels of Evidence: Rating System for the Hierarchy of Evidence

Assessing Level of Evidence	Source of Evidence
Level I	Evidence from a systematic review or meta-analysis of all relevant randomized controlled trials (RCTs) or evidence-based clinical practice guidelines based on systematic reviews of RCTs
Level II	Evidence obtained from at least one well-designed RCT
Level III	Evidence obtained from well-designed controlled trials without randomization (e.g., quasiexperimental study)
Level IV	Evidence from nonexperimental studies (e.g., case-control and cohort studies)
Level V	Evidence from systematic reviews of descriptive and qualitative studies
Level VI	Evidence from a single descriptive or qualitative study
Level VII	Evidence from the opinion of authorities and/or reports of expert committees

(Modified from Melnyk and Fineout-Overholt, 2005.)

1. Review the Koniak-Griffin et al. (2003) article in Appendix A of the text. Then select the appropriate level of evidence category for this study, Level I through Level VII.

2. Review the Davison et al. (2003) article in Appendix D of the text. Then select the appropriate level of evidence category for this study.

POST-TEST

1. Identify whether the following studies are (E) experimental, or (Q) quasiexperimental.

   a. _____ Fifty teen mothers are randomly assigned into an experimental parenting support group and a regular support group. Before the program and at the end of the 3-month program, mother-child interaction patterns are compared between the two groups.

b. _____ Patients on two separate units are given a patient satisfaction with care questionnaire to complete at the end of their first hospital day and on the day of discharge. The patients on one unit receive care directed by a nurse case manager, and the patients on the other unit receive care from the usual rotation of nurses. Patient satisfaction scores are compared.

c. _____ Students are randomly assigned to two groups. One group receives an experimental independent study program and the other receives the usual classroom instruction. Both groups receive the same post-test to evaluate learning.

d. _____ A study was conducted to compare the effectiveness of a music relaxation program with silent relaxation on lowering blood pressure ratings. Subjects were randomly assigned into groups and blood pressures were measured before, during, and immediately after the relaxation exercises.

e. _____ Reading and language development skills were compared between a group of children with chronic otitis media and a group of children without a history of ear problems.

2. Identify the type of experimental or quasiexperimental design for each of the following examples. Use the numbers from the key provided.

   Key: 1 = After-only
   2 = After-only nonequivalent control group
   3 = True experiment
   4 = Nonequivalent control group
   5 = Time series
   6 = Solomon four-group

   a. _____ Nurses are randomly assigned to a new self-study program or the usual ECG teaching program. Knowledge of ECGs is tested before and after the program for both groups.

   b. _____ Babies who tested positive on toxicology screening at birth are randomly assigned into groups to either receive routine care or to receive a special public health nurse intervention program. Health outcomes are tested and compared at 6 months.

   c. _____ A school nurse clinic is set up at one school. Health care outcomes are measured at the end of a year from that school and compared with health outcomes at a comparable school that does not have a clinic.

d. _____ Diabetic patients were randomly assigned to either one of two control groups receiving routine home health care or to one of two groups with a new diabetic teaching program. Patients in one of the control groups and in one of the teaching groups took a test of diabetic knowledge as soon as they were assigned to a group. Patients in the other two groups were not pretested. All patients completed a post-test at the conclusion of the 3-week program.

e. _____ A new peer AIDS prevention program was implemented in one high school. A second high school without the program served as a control group. An AIDS knowledge test was administered at both schools before and after the program was completed.

f. _____ Trends in patient falls were summarized each week one year before and for the first year after implementation of a new hospital-based quality assurance program.

Please check with your instructor for the answers to the post-test.

REFERENCES

Barkauskas VH, Lusk SL, Eakin BL (2005). Selecting control interventions for clinical outcome studies, *West J Nurs Res* 27(3):346-363.

Davison BJ, Goldenberg SL, Gleave ME, et al. (2003). Provision of individualized information to men and their partners to facilitate treatment decision making in prostate cancer, *Oncol Nurs Forum* 30(1):107-114.

Heye JL, Foster L, Bartlett MK, et al. (2002). A preoperative intervention for pain reduction, improved mobility, and self-efficacy, *Appl Nurs Res* 15(3):174-183.

Hoskins S, Coleman M, McNeely D (2005). Stress in carers of individuals with dementia and community mental health teams: An uncontrolled evaluation study, *J Adv Nurs* 50(3):325-333.

Koniak-Griffin D, Verzemnieks IL, Anderson NLR, et al. (2003). Nurse visitation for adolescent mothers: Two-year infant health and maternal outcomes, *Nurs Res* 52(2):127-136.

L'Herault J, Petroff L, Jeffrey J (2001). The effectiveness of a thermal mattress in stabilizing and maintaining body temperature during the transport of very low-birth weight newborns, *Appl Nurs Res* 14(4):210-219.

Melnyk BM, Fineout-Overholt E (2005). Rapid critical appraisal of randomized controlled trials (RCTs): An essential skill for evidence-based practice (EBP), *Pediatr Nurs* 31(1):50-52.

White-Traut RC, Berbaum ML, Lessen B, et al. (2005). Feeding readiness in preterm infants: The relationship between preterm behavioral state and feeding readiness behaviors and efficiency during transition from gavage to oral feeding, *MCN Am J Matern Child Nurs* 30(1):52-59.

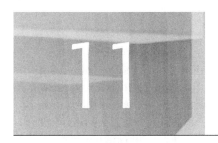

Nonexperimental Designs

INTRODUCTION

Nonexperimental designs can provide extensive amounts of data that can help fill in the gaps found in nursing research. These designs help us clarify, see the real world, and assess relationships between variables, and they can provide clues to direct future, more controlled research. In this way, experimental, quasiexperimental, and nonexperimental designs complement each other. Each provides necessary components of our knowledge base. Nonexperimental designs allow us to discover some of the territory of nursing knowledge before trying to rearrange parts of it. It can be the base on which knowledge is built and further refined with quasiexperimental and experimental research.

LEARNING OUTCOMES

On completion of this chapter, the student should be able to do the following:

- Describe the overall purpose of nonexperimental designs.
- Describe the characteristics of survey, relationship, and difference designs.
- Define the differences among survey, relationship, and difference designs.
- List the advantages and disadvantages of surveys and each type of relationship and difference designs.
- Identify methodological, secondary analysis, and meta-analysis types of research.
- Identify the purposes of methodological, secondary analysis, and meta-analysis types of research.
- Discuss relational inferences versus causal inferences as they relate to nonexperimental designs.
- Identify the criteria used to critique nonexperimental research designs.
- Apply the critiquing criteria to the evaluation of nonexperimental research designs as they appear in research reports.
- Apply levels of evidence to nonexperimental designs.

Activity 1

Determine an answer for each of the following items. Once you have an answer, study the diagram to find each answer. The words will always be in a straight line. They may be read up or down, left to right, right to left, or diagonally. When you find one of the words, draw a circle around it. Any single letter may be used in more than one word, but when the puzzle is finished, not all words will be used. There are no spaces or hyphens between the words in the puzzle, thus if it is a multiword answer, link the letters together as if it is all one word. Some of the terms will be used more than once to fill in the blanks in the statements below.

Experimental Design Puzzle

```
L O N G I T U D I N A L D M E
C I S P U E Q W H X O I Y H X
C R F L G Y Q E R C X E C G P
U W O L Z S B Q F H V O H H O
N T L S C I S Z A R R O I U S
L G T R S D L D U R Z L D O T
U E I O I S Q S E D L V W O F
I U W S J J E L O S Y U H I A
G T D K X O A C I E M D I I C
Q W R E E T O K T T E S T A T
A S A M I K E N B I B H U L O
D U O O K L H N P H O B Z V F
M C N G U L U E O L Y N R K C
K A M F G U P Q S B Z L A H T
L W J F V N E W J S W L E L V
```

1. This type is better known for the breadth than the depth of data collected. _____

2. A major disadvantage is the length of time needed for data collection. _____

3. The main question is whether or not variables covary. _____

4. These words mean *after the fact.* _____

5. This eliminates the confounding variable of maturation. _____

6. This quantifies the magnitude and direction of a relationship. _____

7. Collects data from the same group at several points in time. _____

8. Can be surprisingly accurate if the sample is representative. _____

9. Uses data from one point in time. _____

10. This is based on two or more naturally occurring groups with different conditions of the presumed independent variable. _____

Activity 2

Listed below are a series of advantages and disadvantages for various types of nonexperimental designs. For each type of design, pick at least one advantage (A) and one disadvantage (D) from the list that accurately describes a quality of the design. Then insert the A or D and the appropriate number in the list below.

	Advantages	Disadvantages
Correlation studies	_____	_____
Cross-sectional	_____	_____
Ex post facto	_____	_____
Longitudinal	_____	_____
Prospective	_____	_____
Retrospective	_____	_____
Survey	_____	_____

Advantages
A1 A great deal of information can be economical obtained from a large population.
A2 Ability to assess changes in the variables of interest over time.
A3 Explores relationship between variables that are inherently not manipulable.
A4 Offers a higher level of control than a correlational study.
A5 They facilitate intelligent decision-making, using objective criteria to guide the process.
A6 Each subject is followed separately and serves as his own control.
A7 Stronger than retrospective studies because of the degree of control on extraneous variables.
A8 Less time-consuming, less expensive, and thus more manageable for the researcher.

Disadvantages
D1 The inability to draw a causal linkage between two variables.
D2 An alternative hypothesis could be the reason for the relationships.
D3 The researcher is unable to manipulate the variables of interest.

D4 The researcher is unable to determine a causal relationship between variables because of lack of manipulation, control, and randomization.

D5 The information obtained tends to be superficial.

D6 The researcher must know sampling techniques, questionnaire construction, interviewing, and data analysis.

D7 No randomization in sampling because studying preexisting groups.

D8 Internal validity threats such as testing and mortality are present.

D9 Subject loss to follow-up and attrition may lead to unintended sample bias that affects external validity and generalizability of findings.

Activity 3

Each of the following are excerpts from nonexperimental studies. For each example, determine the type of design utilized from the list provided. Not all designs are used as examples, and some will be used more than once.

C	Correlation studies
CS	Cross-sectional
E	Ex post facto
L	Longitudinal
M	Methodological
MA	Meta-analysis
P	Prospective
R	Retrospective
SC	Survey comparative
SD	Survey descriptive
SE	Survey exploratory

Remember, some studies use more than one type of nonexperimental design.

1. Van Cleve et al. (2004) (Appendix B of the text) conducted a study to describe children's pain for 1 year after their diagnosis of acute lymphatic leukemia, to study strategies used by children and their families to manage pain associated with lymphocytic leukemia, and to examine the outcomes of management effectiveness and functional status. The researchers collected data at seven data points from 95 English- and Spanish-speaking children, ages 4 to 17 years. Age-appropriate instruments were used to examine the variables.

   Type of design:

2. To identify factors that influence American and Icelandic parents' health perceptions, parents in these two countries who had children aged 6 years or younger with chronic asthma completed questionnaires regarding family demands, caregiving demands, family hardiness, sense of coherence, and health perceptions. Data were collected from 76 Ameri-

can families and 103 Icelandic families who signed a consent form and then were given a package of questionnaires by mail or in person. If they did not respond in 14 days they received a follow-up phone call. (Svavarsdóttir and Rayens 2003)

Type of design:

3. Two groups of high-risk Medicaid-eligible mothers were compared. One group (n=21) participated in a maternal home visitation program while the second group (N=198) did not. All mothers were interviewed in their homes using structured, face-to-face interviews. Data collection occurred once during pregnancy and once approximately one year after delivery. (Navaie-Waliser et al. 2001)

Type of design:

4. One hundred-twenty RNs who worked in critical care or step-down units completed the Handwashing Assessment Inventory (HAI). The consent form and the HAI were mailed to RNs who agreed to participate. A stamped, self-addressed envelope was included so the RNs could return the completed material to the investigators. (O'Boyle et al. 2001)

Type of design:

5. The level of depressive symptoms experienced by women was measured in association with resource availability, exposure to risk factors, and intrinsic strength factors. Three questionnaires were completed by 315 women of Mexican descent living in an urban community in northern California. (Heilelmann et al. 2002)

Type of design:

6. Twenty-three items were initially developed for the Atkins Osteoporosis Risk Assessment Tool (ORAT) after a thorough examination of the literature. These items were reviewed for relevance to the domain of content by a panel of eight experts using Lynn's (1986) two-stage process for content validation. (Wynd and Schaefer 2002)

Type of design:

7. The purpose of this study is to clarify the concept of social support. The Template Verification and Expansion Model of concept development were used in this study. An electronic search of the literature in several databases (CINAHL, MEDLINE, PsycINFO, and Soc Abs) was conducted to find qualitative studies and linguistic analyses of the concept of social support. The 44 qualitative studies and 3 linguistic analyses of social support were included in this study. (Finfgeld-Conett 2005)

Type of Design:

Activity 4

Use the critiquing criteria from the chapter to analyze the following excerpt from a study.

In a 1997 article by Mohr, her objective was: "This study is the context portion of a larger study that described the experience of 30 nurses in Texas, USA who worked in for-profit psychiatric hospitals during a documented period of corporate deviance. The objective of the contextual portion was to describe the major findings in 1991-1992 of investigating agencies that probed the scandal" (p. 39). The sample consisted of over 1,240 pages and 40 hours of corporate records obtained under subpoena, and written and oral testimony before the U.S. House Select Committee on Children, Youth, and Families.

1. Type of design:

The findings were four themes: insurance games, dumping patients, patient abuse, and playing with the language.

   The conclusions: "Organizational deviance may become more widespread in profit-driven systems of care. Lobbying for whistleblower protection, collective advocacy, and creative educational reforms are used" are presented in the frontpiece of the article. However, under the "Discussion and Recommendations" section, the author states: "As suggested by social scientists, research can serve as the basis for reflection, critique, and action... For example, because nurses are professionals who have a special contract with the public and are concerned with health teaching and promotion, they might implement counter-hegemonic activity by collective advocacy and criticizing information distortion."

2. Does the research go beyond the relational parameters of the findings and erroneously infer cause-and-effect relationships between the variables? (Circle the correct answer.)

   Yes   No   (If yes, explain below.)

Activity 5

Review the Critical Thinking Decision Path: Nonexperimental Design Choice found in the textbook. If you wanted to test a relationship between two variables in the past such as the incidence of reported back injuries of nurses working in newborn nursery compared with those nurses working in long-term care, which design would you use?

Activity 6: Web-Based Activity

This activity will assist you in finding nursing research survey instruments if you are considering gathering data for a nonexperimental survey study. Use two search engines (Google, Google Scholar) and one website (PubMed) to find instruments, and then compare the three sources to determine which is the most helpful to you.

1. First, go to the National Library of Medicine, PubMed site at http://www.pubmed.gov.

   You will see a box labeled "Search" with the term "PubMed" in it. The box next to it has the label "for" before it; type in "Nursing Research Survey Instruments." Click on Go. Review the results you obtain.

   a. How many results were identified?

   b. Print the first page and review the first five citations. Do these citations give you information about the survey instruments that are available to use in nursing research?

   c. How is the information presented? Is it in a manner that is useful to planning research?

   d. How current is the information?

2. Now go to the website http://www.google.com. In the box, type in "Nursing Research Survey Instruments." Click on "Google Search." Review the results you obtain.

   a. How many results were identified?

   b. Print the first page and review the first five citations. Do these citations give you information about the survey instruments that are available to use in nursing research?

   c. How is the information presented? Is it in a manner that is useful to planning research?

   d. How current is the information?

3. Now go to the website http://scholar.google.com. In the box, type "Nursing Research Survey Instruments." Click on "Search." Review the results you obtain.

   a. How many results were identified?

   b. Print the first page and review the first five citations. Do these citations give you information about the survey instruments that are available to use in nursing research?

c. How is the information presented? Is it in a manner that is useful to planning research?

d. How current is the information?

☀ Activity 7: Evidence-Based Practice Activity

1. What is the value of nonexperimental studies, such as ones that demonstrate a strong relationship in predictive correlational studies for evidence-based practice?
   a. None
   b. They provide evidence only for training purposes.
   c. They demonstrate cause-and-effect relationships and can be utilized in decision-making regarding changes in practice.
   d. They lend support for attempting to influence the independent variable in a future intervention study.

2. Which of the following nonexperimental designs provides a quality of evidence for evidence-based practice that is stronger than the others, because the researcher can determine the incidence of a problem and its possible causes?
   a. Cross-sectional
   b. Longitudinal cohort
   c. Survey

3. When you, the research consumer, are using the evidence-based practice model to consider a change in practice, you will initially make your decision based on the strength and quality of evidence provided by the meta-analysis. Following this, what other two characteristics will be important for you to consider? (There are two correct responses.)
   a. Clinical expertise
   b. Patient values
   c. The strength of the evidence
   d. The quality of the evidence
   e. The literature review

POST-TEST

Choose from among the following words to complete the post-test. Each word may be used one time; however, this list duplicates some words because they are used in more than one answer.

Comparative	Exploratory	Methodological	Retrospective
Correlational	Ex post facto	Prospective	Retrospective
Cross-sectional	Interrelational	Prospective	Survey
Cross-sectional	Longitudinal	Relationship-difference	Variables
Descriptive	Longitudinal	Retrospective	

1. In comparative surveys, the researcher does not manipulate the
    _____ but assesses data in order to provide data for future nursing intervention studies

2. _____ is the broadest category of nonexperimental design.

3. The category from item #2 can be further classified as _____, _____, and _____.

4. The second major category of nonexperimental design according to LoBiondo-Wood and Haber includes _____ studies.

5. The researcher is using _____ design when examining the relationship between two or more variables.

6. _____ designs have many similarities to quasiexperimental designs.

7. _____ design used in epidemiological work is similar to ex post facto.

8. LoBiondo-Wood and Haber discuss three types of developmental studies. They are:
    a.

    b.

    c.

9. _____ studies collect data at one point in time while _____ collects data from the same group at different points in time.

10. A(n)_____ study looks at presumed causes and moves forward in time to presumed effects.

11. The researcher is using a _____ design if he or she is trying to link present events to events that have occurred in the past.

12. The _____ researcher is interested in identifying an intangible construct (concept) and making it tangible with a paper-and-pencil instrument or observation protocol.

Please check with your instructor for the answers to the post-test.

REFERENCES

Finfgeld-Conett D (2005). Clarification of social support, *J of Nurs Schol* 31(1):4-9.

Heilelmann MV, Lee KA, Kury FS (2002). Strengths and vulnerabilities of women of Mexican descent in relation to depressive symptoms, *Nurs Res* 51(3):175-182.

Mohr WK (1997). Outcomes of corporate greed, *Image: J Nurs Schol* 29:39-45.

Navaie-Waliser M, Martin SL, Tessaro I, et al. (2001). Social support and psychological functioning among high-risk mothers: The impact of Baby Love Maternal Outreach Worker Program, *Public Health Nursing* 17(4):280-291.

O'Boyle CA, Henly SJ, Duckett LJ (2001). Nurses' motivation to wash their hands: A standardized measurement approach, *Appl Nurs Res* 14(3):136-145.

Svavarsdóttir EK, Rayens MK (2003). American and Icelandic parents' perceptions of the health status of their young children with chronic asthma, *Image: J of Nurs Schol* 35(4): 351-358.

Van Cleve L, Bossert E, Beecroft P, et al. (2004). The pain experience of children with leukemia during the first year after diagnosis, *Nurs Res* 53(1):1-10.

Wynd CA, Schaefer MA (2002). The osteoporosis risk assessment tool: Establishing content validity through a panel of experts, *Appl Nurs Res* 16(2):184-188.

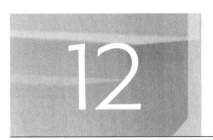

Sampling

INTRODUCTION

Sampling is a process of selection in which individuals, objects, animals, or events are chosen to represent the population of a study. The ideal sampling strategy is one in which the elements truly represent the population being studied while controlling for any source of bias. The specific research question(s) determines the selection of the sample, variables to measure, and a sampling frame. The sampling strategies are important and should enable the choice of a sample that represents the target population and controls for bias as much as possible to ensure that the research will be valid. Reality modulates the ideal with the consideration of sampling in relation to efficiency, practicality, ethics, and availability of subjects, which can alter the ideal strategy for a given study.

LEARNING OUTCOMES

On completion of this chapter, the student should be able to do the following:

- Identify the purpose of sampling.
- Define the population, sample, and sampling.
- Compare and contrast a population and a sample.
- Discuss the eligibility criteria for sample selection.
- Define nonprobability and probability sampling.
- Identify the types of nonprobability and probability sampling strategies.
- Compare the advantages and disadvantages of specific nonprobability and probability sampling strategies.
- Discuss the contribution of nonprobability and probability sampling strategies to strength of evidence provided by study findings.
- Discuss the factors that influence determination of sample size.
- Discuss the procedure for drawing a sample.
- Identify the criteria for critiquing a sampling plan.
- Use the critiquing criteria to evaluate the "Sample" section of a research report.

Activity 1

Identify the category of sampling for each of the following sampling strategies. Use the abbreviations from the key provided.

Key:
P = Probability sampling
N = Nonprobability sampling

1. _____   Convenience sampling

2. _____   Purposive sampling

3. _____   Simple random sampling

4. _____   Quota sampling

5. _____   Cluster sampling

6. _____   Systematic sampling

7. _____   Stratified random sampling

Activity 2

For each of the following examples of studies, identify the sampling strategy used from the following list. Write a letter that corresponds to the strategy in the space preceding the sampling description. Check the glossary for definition of terms.

   a. Convenience sampling
   b. Quota sampling
   c. Purposive sampling
   d. Simple random sampling
   e. Stratified random sampling
   f. Systematic sampling

1. _____   The sample for the study of critical thinking behavior of undergraduate baccalaureate nursing students consisted of students enrolled in junior- and senior-level courses in three specific schools of nursing. In each program, students are invited to participate until a total sample representing 10% of the junior-level students and 10% of the senior-level students was obtained.

2. _____   Every eighth person on the diabetic clinic patient roster was asked to participate in the study. A table of random numbers was used to select the beginning of the sampling within the first sampling interval.

3. _____   Using a table of random numbers, the sample of 50 subjects was selected from a list of all mothers giving birth in the county during the first 6 months of the year.

4. _____ The sample was selected from residents of eight nursing homes in Arkansas and consisted of cognitively impaired people with no physical impairments or other psychiatric illness.

5. _____ The sample selected was parents who were chosen because of their knowledge and experience of having been a parent with a child in a NICU. Inclusion criteria included those parents with a child: admitted to the NICU for more than a week, gestation at birth 26 weeks or above, on a ventilator for at least 3 days, and discharged home within the last 6 months.

6. _____ The sample consisted of adolescent mothers, meeting eligibility requirements, who were recruited from referrals to the Community Health Services Division of the County Health Department until the sample reached a target number of 144 participants. The mothers were randomly assigned using a computer-based program into one of two groups.

7. _____ To study the educational opportunities for nurses in various ethnic groups, a list of all nurses in the state of California was sorted by ethnicity. The sample consisted of 10% of the nurses in each ethnic group, selected according to a table of random numbers.

8. _____ A total of 155 infants were enrolled and divided into an intervention group of 72 infants and a control group of 83 infants. The numerical assignment was based on the weight and gestational age.

Activity 3

1. Refer to the study by Davison et al. (2003) in Appendix D of your textbook.

   a. Is the sample adequately described?
   Yes   No

   b. Do the sample characteristics correspond to the larger population?
   Yes   No   Maybe

   c. What sampling strategy was used in this study?

   d. Is this a probability or nonprobability sample?

   e. Is the sample size appropriate?
   Yes   No   Unsure

2. List one advantage of using the sampling strategy described in this study.

3. List one disadvantage of using the sampling strategy described in this study.

4. How does this sampling strategy support evidence in nursing practice?

Activity 4

Using the critical thinking decision path in the textbook, indicate whether the following statements are True (T) or False (F).

1. _____   Nonprobability sampling is associated with less generalizability to the larger population.

2. _____   Convenience sampling limits generalizability of findings largely because of the self-selection of subjects.

3. _____   Nonprobability sampling strategies are more time-consuming than probability strategies.

4. _____   Random sampling has the greatest risk of bias and is moderately representative.

5. _____   The easier the sampling strategy the greater the risk of bias, and as sampling becomes easier to implement, the risk of bias and limited representatives of the population increases.

6. _____   Purposive sampling procedures are the least generalizable sampling of the sampling strategies listed.

7. _____   Stratified random sampling uses a random selection procedure for obtaining sample subjects.

Activity 5

Review the following excerpt from a study. Using the critiquing criteria listed in the text, critique the sampling process used in this study. Refer to the study by Van Cleve et al. (2004) in Appendix B of your text.

The sample of 95 English- and Spanish-speaking children, ages 4 to 17 years with acute lymphocytic leukemia who were receiving care in one of three southern California hospitals participated in the interviews for this study. The subjects were invited to participate if they were within one month of diagnosis and either English- or Spanish-speaking. The questions in the interview were directed to the child, with supplemental responses from the parent. There were 48 Latino subjects, 32 of whom were Spanish-speaking. The remaining 16 chose to respond in English.

The data reflected the demographics of the three counties in which the facilities were located. The sample of 95 children provided a broad representation of age groups, gender, ethnic groups, and treatment protocols. Pain intensity scores incorporated the following responses: children 4 to 7 years old, the highest and lowest mean scores, respectively, were 2 and 1.6 (scale, 0-4). For the children 8 to 17 years old, the highest and lowest mean scores, respectively, were 50.1 and 39.5 (scale, 0-100). The most common location of pain was the legs (26.5%) in all seven interviews. Other frequently noted sites were the abdomen (16.6%), and back (14.2%). Age-appropriate instruments were used to examine the variables of pain intensity, location pattern over time, perceived effectiveness of management strategies, and functional status.

According to the interviews, the most frequently used strategy for pain management was stressor modification (e.g., medication, sleep, hot/cold, and massage). The most common coping strategies according to a Likert scale were "watch TV," "lie down," "wish it would go away," or "tell my mother or father."

1. Have the sample characteristics been completely described? (Explain your answer.)

2. Can the parameters of the study population be inferred from the description of the sample?

3. To what extent is the sample representative of the population as defined?

4. Are criteria for eligibility in the sample specifically identified?

5. Have sample delimitations been established? (Explain your answer.)

6. Would it be possible to replicate the study sample? (Explain your answer.)

7. How was the sample selected? Is the method of sample selection appropriate?

8. What kind of bias, if any, is introduced by this method?

9. Is the sample size appropriate? How is it substantiated?

10. Are there indications that the rights of the subjects have been ensured?

11. Do the researchers identify the limitations in generalizability of the findings from the sample to the population? Are they appropriate?

12. Do the researchers indicate how replication of the study with other samples would provide increased support for the findings?

Activity 6: Web-Based Activity

Go to the U.S. Census website at http://www.census.gov. Click on "Find an Area Profile with Quick Facts" at the bottom right-hand corner of the screen. In the box where it asks you, "To begin, select a state from this list or use the map to your right," select California from the drop down menu. Click on the "Go" button.

1. Under California Quick Facts, look at the item titled: "White persons, percent 2000" and write down that percent.

2. Now look for the item titled: "Persons of Hispanic or Latino origin, percent 2000." Write down that percent for California.

3. What age groups do these percents include?

4. Now go back to Activity 5. Are the sample percents in the Van Cleve et al. (2004) study for White and Hispanic people the same as they are for Hispanic and Whites in the 2000 census data for the state of California? Would the sample percents for Hispanic and Whites in the Van Cleve et al. study be representative of the population of California?

☼ Activity 7: Evidence-Based Practice Activity

The text defines evidence-based practice (EBP) as the integration of best research evidence with clinical expertise and patient values. EBP allows nurses to utilize research findings to make decisions to improve practice. Teams of nurses are applying multiple study findings to improve practice outcomes with individuals, families, and other healthcare professionals. Through this practice, more effective patient teaching and quality care are being realized.

What is the relationship between sampling and evidence-based practice decision-making? In other words, how will the sampling strategy in a study or a meta-analysis of studies influence how you and your colleagues make a decision about changing the practice in your health care setting? (Hint: Review the five Evidence-Based Practice Tips in chapter 12 before answering this question.)

POST-TEST

Complete the sentences below.

1. A statistical technique known as _____ may be used to determine sample size in quantitative studies.

2. Sampling strategies are grouped into two categories: _____ sampling and _____ sampling.

3. _____ sampling is the use of the most readily accessible people or objects as subjects in a study.

4. Advantages of _____ sampling are low bias and maximal representativeness, but the disadvantage is the labor in drawing a sample.

5. A(n) _____ can be used to select an unbiased sample or unbiased assignment of subjects to treatment groups.

6. A(n) _____ sample is one whose key characteristics closely approximate those of the population.

7. _____ criteria are used to select the sample from all possible units and _____ may be used to restrict the population to a homogenous group of subjects.

8. Types of nonprobability sampling include _____, _____, and _____ sampling.

9. Successive random sampling of units that progress from large to small and meet sample eligibility criteria is known as _____ sampling.

10. In certain qualitative studies, subjects are added to the sample until _____ occurs (new data no longer emerge during data collection).

Please check with your instructor for the answers to the post-test.

REFERENCES

Davison BJ, Goldenberg SL, Gleave ME, et al. (2003). Provision of individualized information to men and their partners to facilitate treatment decision making in prostate cancer, *Oncol Nurs Forum* 30(1):107-114.

U.S. Census Bureau. Accessed July 21, 2005 from http://www.census.gov.

Van Cleve L, Bossert E, Beecroft P, et al. (2004). The pain experience of children with leukemia during the first year after diagnosis, *Nurs Res* 53(1):1-10.

Legal and Ethical Issues

INTRODUCTION

Patient advocacy is one of the primary roles of a professional nurse. Nowhere is this more important than in the field of research. The nurse must be a patient advocate, whether acting as the researcher, a participant in data gathering, a provider of care for research subjects, or a research consumer. A multitude of legal and ethical issues exist in research; nurses must be aware of, assess, act on, and evaluate these issues. In addition, nurses need to be knowledgeable about the purpose and functions of the institutional review board (IRB) and the federal regulations on which they are based.

LEARNING OUTCOMES

On completion of this chapter, the student should be able to do the following:

- Describe the historical background that led to the development of ethical guidelines for the use of human subjects in research.
- Identify the essential elements of an informed consent form.
- Evaluate the adequacy of an informed consent form.
- Describe the institutional review board's role in the research review process.
- Identify populations of subjects who require special legal and ethical research considerations.
- Appreciate the nurse researcher's obligations to conduct and report research in an ethical manner.
- Describe the nurse's role as patient advocate in research situations.
- Discuss the nurse's role in ensuring that FDA guidelines for testing of medical devices are followed.
- Discuss animal rights in research situations.
- Critique the ethical aspects of a research study.

Activity 1

Fill in the blanks with the correct term from the following list (you do not need to use all of the terms):

Beneficence   Justice
Confidentiality   Nursing research committee
Expedited review   Unauthorized research
Institutional review board   Unethical research study
HIPAA

1. _____ reviews proposals for scientific merit and congruence with the institutional policies and missions.

2. _____ reviews research proposals to assure protection of the rights of human subjects.

3. The idea that human subjects should be treated fairly and should not be denied a benefit to which the subject is entitled is _____.

4. A study of existing data that is of minimal risk to subjects may be a candidate for a(n) _____.

5. The U.S. Public Health Service studied the effects of untreated syphilis on African-American sharecroppers in Tuskegee, Alabama and withheld penicillin treatment even after penicillin was commonly available. This is considered a(n) _____.

6. Regulation requires the healthcare profession to protect privacy of patient information and create standards for electronic data exchange _____.

Activity 2

List the three ethical principles relevant to the conduct of research involving human subjects. These were included in the Belmont Report (1979) and formed the basis for regulations affecting research sponsored by the federal government.

1.

2.

3.

Activity 3

Read the following example of a Research Consent form. Then review the list of the elements of informed consent that follows the example. For each item in the list of elements of informed consent, put either a "√" if the element is included in the consent or a "0" if it is absent from the consent. Summarize your findings in a paragraph at the end of the exercise.

Research Consent Form
Agreement to Participate in Research

Responsible Investigator: Mary Jo Gorney-Moreno, PhD, Professor, Nursing

Title of Protocol: A web-based interactive program to engage nurses in learning principles of pain management.

We are recruiting nursing students to test a web-based interactive program to engage nurses in learning principles of pain management. There are three learning outcomes for this program, to teach: (1) appropriate and safe control of the patient's pain, (2) prevention and management of side effects of pain management, and (3) to provide accurate and complete patient teaching regarding pain and side effect management. At the end of the simulation, you will receive 3 scores, one for how well you managed patient care in each of these areas. It will take about 30 minutes to complete the simulation. The simulation is available online at http://www.cdl.edu/painless. You can complete the simulation as many times as you like; each time you will be presented with a new set of variables for the patient, Mr. Sanchez. The variables are programmed to appear randomly. We hope that this activity will enhance your knowledge related to providing pain management for your patients. There are no known risks for participation.

If you agree to participate, we welcome you and would like you to complete a pre- and post-test, as well as a short evaluation form after you complete the simulation. Your participation is voluntary, and you may withdraw at any time and for any reason. There is no penalty for not participating or withdrawing. The personal benefits for participation include assisting faculty and yourself to understand more about the effectiveness of this innovative educational intervention and to increase your knowledge. There are no costs to you or any other party.

I will ask you to print a copy of your scores from the simulation, and complete the pre- and post-test and a short questionnaire. All data collected will be coded using a unique five-character string and will not be identified with you personally. There is no risk to you.

Dr. Mary Jo Gorney-Moreno, Professor, School of Nursing, San Jose State University is conducting this study. Dr. Gorney-Moreno can be reached at 408-555-1000. You should understand that your participation is voluntary and that choosing not to participate in this study, or in any part of this study, will not affect your relations with San Jose State University. You may refuse to participate in the entire study or in any part of the study; you are free to withdraw at any time without any negative effect on your relations with San Jose State University. The results of this study may be published, but any information that could result in your identification will remain confidential. If you have questions about this study, I will be happy to talk with you. I can be reached at

---

408-555-1000. If you have questions or complaints about research subjects' rights, or in the event of a research-related injury, please contact Serena Smith, PhD, Associate Vice President for Graduate Studies and Research, at (408) 555-1000.

This project has been reviewed and approved according to the San Jose State University Human Subjects Institutional Review Board procedures governing human subjects research.

Your signature indicates that you have been fully informed of your rights and voluntarily agree to participate in this study. You will be given a copy of this signed form.

By signing this form, I agree to participate in this study.

_____   _____
Subject's Signature   Date

Elements of Informed Consent

1. _____   Title of protocol
2. _____   Invitation to participate
3. _____   Basis for subject selection
4. _____   Overall purpose of the study
5. _____   Explanation of benefits
6. _____   Description of risks and discomforts
7. _____   Potential benefits
8. _____   Alternatives to participation
9. _____   Financial obligations
10. _____   Assurance of confidentiality
11. _____   In case of injury compensation
12. _____   HIPAA disclosure
13. _____   Subject withdrawal
14. _____   Offer to answer questions
15. _____   Concluding consent statement
16. _____   Identification of investigators

Activity 4

Nurses must be aware of populations who require special legal and ethical considerations. List at least four groups of subjects who are vulnerable or have diminished autonomy and thus require extra protection as research subjects.

1.

2.

3.

4.

Activity 5

Match the violation of ethical principle described from the following list with the examples presented below. More than one violation may have occurred in the examples that are cited. List all that were violated.

    a. Degree of risk outweighed benefits
    b. Subjects not informed they could withdraw from study at any time
    c. Subjects not informed or offered the effective treatment that was available
    d. Lack of informed consent
    e. No evidence of IRB approval prior to start of research
    f. Right to fair treatment and protection
    g. Principles of informed consent violated or incomplete disclosure of potential risk, harm, results or side effects was not given

1. Write the letter(s) describing violation after the description of the study.

    UCLA Schizophrenic Medication Study—A 1983 study examining the effects of withdrawing psychotropic medications of 50 patients under treatment for schizophrenia. Twenty-three subjects suffered severe relapses after their medications were stopped. The goal of the study was to determine if some schizophrenics might do better without medications that had deleterious side effects. Patients were not informed that their symptoms could worsen or about the severity of a potential relapse. _____

2. List the letter(s) that corresponds to the ethical violation(s) listed.

    The United States Public Health Service conducted a study from 1932-1973 on two groups of poor African-American male sharecroppers. One group had untreated syphilis and the other did not. Treatment was withheld from the group diagnosed with syphilis, even after it became generally available and known to be effective. Steps were taken to prevent infected subjects from obtaining penicillin. The researchers wanted to study the effects of untreated syphilis. _____

Activity 6

This activity assesses the utilization of procedures for protecting basic human rights. Review the articles in Appendices A through D of the text. For each article, describe how informed consent was obtained, and whether the author described obtaining permission from the institutional review board.

1. Koniak-Griffin et al. (2003):

2. Van Cleve et al. (2004):

3. Plach et al. (2004):

4. Davison et al. (2003):

Activity 7: Web-Based Activity

Go to the website http://www.cancer.gov.

1. Identify the source of this website. _____

2. Is this a reputable source that would provide reliable and valid information to inform a nursing practice?

   Yes, because _____

   No, because _____

Click on "Clinical Trials" at the top. Scroll down and click on "Conducting Clinical Trials." At the left, select "Participants in Clinical Trials," then click on the link "Human Participant Protections Education for Research Teams." Fill in the registration information with a username and password of your choice. Review the tutorial and complete the online quiz to determine your comprehension of this material. The NIH now requires education in the protection of human research participants for all investigators and key personnel submitting NIH applications for grants or proposals for contracts, or receiving new or noncompeting awards. You may complete this program if you like, or if your instructor requires it. If you complete all the tutorials successfully, print the certificate and add this item to your résumé.

☀ Activity 8: Evidence-Based Practice Activity

You are a nurse working in a postpartum unit. If you decided to make a change in your practice based on an evidence-based practice article, but first wanted to check to be certain that no misconduct had occurred in the conduct or reporting of the study, where would you find this information?

POST-TEST

1. It is necessary for researchers and nurses to protect the basic human rights of vulnerable groups. Can research studies be conducted with these populations?

   Yes, because _____

   No, because _____

2. A researcher must receive IRB approval (before, after) beginning to conduct research involving humans.

3. If you question whether a researcher has permission to conduct a study in your hospital, which documents would you want to see that demonstrate approval from which group(s)?

   _____

4. Should a researcher list all the possible risks and benefits of a participating in a research study even if some people may refuse because these items are listed in detail?

   Yes   No

5. If you agreed to collect data for a researcher who had not asked the patient's permission to participate in the research study, you would be violating the patient's right to

   _____.

6. What are two of the risks of scientific fraud or misconduct? _____

   _____

Please check with your instructor for the answers to the post-test.

REFERENCES

Davison BJ, Goldenberg SL, Gleave ME, et al. (2003). Provision of individualized information to men and their partners to facilitate treatment decision making in prostate cancer, *Oncol Nurs Forum* 30(1):107-114.

Koniak-Griffin D, Verzemnieks IL, Anderson NLR, et al. (2003). Nurse visitation for adolescent mothers: Two-year infant health and maternal outcomes, *Nurs Res* 52(2):127-136.

National Cancer Institute. Accessed September 1, 2005 from http://www.cancer.gov.

Plach SK, Stevens PE, Moss VA (2004). Social role experiences of women living with rheumatoid arthritis, *J Family Nurs* 10(1):33-49.

Van Cleve L, Bossert E, Beecroft P, et al. (2004). The pain experience of children with leukemia during the first year after diagnosis, *Nurs Res* 53(1):1-10.

14 Data-Collection Methods

INTRODUCTION

> Observe, probe
> Details unfold
> Let nature's secrets
> Be stammeringly retold.
> —Goethe

The focus of this chapter is basic information about data collection. As a consumer of research, the reader needs the skills to evaluate and critique data-collection methods in published research studies. In order to achieve these skills, it is helpful to have an appreciation of the process or the critical thinking "journey" the researcher has taken to be ready to collect the data. Each of the preceding chapters represented important preliminary steps in the research planning and designing phases prior to data collection. Although most researchers are eager to begin data collection, the planning for data collection is very important. The planning includes identifying and prioritizing data needs, developing or selecting appropriate data collection tools, and selecting and training data-collection personnel before proceeding with actual collection of data.

The five types of data-collection methods differ in their basic approach and the strengths and weaknesses of their characteristics. Readers should be prepared to ask questions about the appropriateness of the measures chosen by the researcher to gather data about the variable of concern. This includes determining the objectivity, consistency, quantifiability, observer intervention, and/or obtrusiveness of the chosen data-collection method.

LEARNING OUTCOMES

On completion of this chapter, the reader should be able to do the following:

- Define the types of data-collection methods used in nursing research.
- List the advantages and disadvantages of each data-collection method.

- Compare how specific data-collection methods contribute to the strength of evidence in a research study
- Critically evaluate the data-collection methods used in published nursing research studies.

Activity 1

Review each of the articles referenced below. Be especially thorough in reading the sections that relate to data-collection methods. Answer the questions in relation to what you understand from the article. For some questions, there may be more than one answer.

Study 1
Koniak-Griffin D, et al. (2003) (in Appendix A of the text).

1. Which data-collection method(s) is/are used in this research study?
   a. A physiological measure
   b. An observational measure
   c. An interview measure
   d. A questionnaire measure
   e. Records of available data

2. In your opinion, what would be the advantage in using this method(s)? What explanation do the investigators provide?

Study 2
Van Cleve, et al. (2004) (in Appendix B of the text).

1. Which data-collection method is used in this research study?
   a. A physiological measure
   b. An observational measure
   c. An interview measure
   d. A questionnaire
   e. Records of available data

2. Rationale for appropriateness of data-collection method:

3. What is your opinion as to the success of the method chosen?

Study 3
Plach et al. (2004) (in Appendix C of the text).

1.   What data-collection method is used in this research study?
     a.   A physiological measure
     b.   An observational measure
     c.   An interview measure
     d.   A questionnaire
     e.   Records of available data

2.   What were the strengths in using this method?

Study 4
Davison et al. (2003) (in Appendix D of the text).

1.   What data-collection method is used in this research study?
     a.   A physiological measure
     b.   An observational measure
     c.   An interview measure
     d.   A questionnaire
     e.   Records of available data

2.   Were there any characteristics of the partner pairs that would raise any questions in your
     mind about the use of these methodologies?

Activity 2

Using the content of chapter 14 in the text, have fun with the word search exercise. Answer the
questions below and find the words in the puzzle.

1.   Baccalaureate prepared nurses are _____ of research.
2.   _____ are those methods that use technical instruments to col-
     lect data about patients' physical, chemical, microbiological, or anatomical status.
3.   _____ is the distortion of data as a result of the observer's pres-
     ence.
4.   _____ are best used when a large response rate and an unbiased
     sample are important.

5. _____ data-collection method is subject to problems of availability, authenticity, and accuracy.

6. _____ measurements are especially useful when there are a finite number of questions to be asked and the questions are clear and specific.

7. Essential in the critique of data-collection methods is the emphasis on the appropriateness, _____, and _____ of the method employed.

8. _____ raises ethical questions (especially informed consent issues); therefore, it is not often used in nursing.

9. _____ _____ is the consistency of observations between two or more observers.

10. _____ is the process of translating the concepts/variables into measurable phenomena.

11. _____ is a format that uses close-ended items, and there are a fixed number of alternative responses.

12. _____ is the method for objective, systematic, and quantitative description of communications and documentary evidence.

13. This exercise is supposed to be _____!

```
D E L I V E R S T A T I S T C S Y E S P A S
S S A C A B I N E T F O R K A Z O S P E I O
I A W O P E R A T I O N A L I Z A T I O N B
G T S N O R N E V E R B Y D N E A U X B T J
N S Y S T E M A T I C A J H T B S D V S E E
I F L I K E R T S C A L E E R R O Y A E R C
F A K S C A L E S N O V N O C A A U L R R T
H C U T A C R A T I M A P V E T P U I V A I
Y T B E B H I R T E M A H V W K I C D A T V
P C O N T E N T A N A L Y S I S P V O T E I
R O Y C B K D S I S R T S A D V A N E I R T
E R E Y O D U G K A T P I B I O I O G O R Y
A V S I B R Q U E S T I O N N A I R E N E C
C I A R E S E A R C H L L R E A C E S O L O
T O B M E X C E L A E O O D A T A C O V I N
I U E A E V A L I D S T G N O S T O O E A S
V N Y E S S I N T E R V I E W S A R F R B U
I H A P P I E N E S S P C A T A G D U N I M
T X C I T E D E L P H I A T O T P S N V L E
Y C E A T U B B S A N D L D O N N M A R I R
Y A B L E A C O N C E A L M E N T O O T T R
A I K E V A L I K E I I A B C O N S U M Y S
```

Activity 3

You are reviewing a study, and concealment is necessary; in other words, there is no other way to collect the data, and the data collected will not have negative consequences for the subject.

1. Name at least one population where concealment is not uncommon.

2. How would you obtain subjects' consent?

3. What is the major reason for using concealment?

Activity 4

You are asked to participate in discussions about impending research in your community. The purpose of the study is to identify the health status, beliefs, practices, preventive services currently known and used, and accessibility/availability of health service needs for the residents of your rural community.

In your critical thinking journey, describe what you would consider in the selection of a data-collection method. Review each method and discuss the pros and cons for choosing a specific data-collection method. State your rationale for your final selection. What would be your thinking about instruments and types?

Activity 5

Using the content of chapter 14 in the textbook, circle the correct response for each question. Some questions will have more than one answer.

1. What is a primary advantage of physiological measures?
    a. The measuring tool never affects the phenomena being measured
    b. It is one of the easiest types of methods to implement
    c. It is unlikely that study participants/subjects can distort the physiological information
    d. Their objectivity, sensitivity, and precision
    e. All of the above

2. Self-report measures are usually more useful than observation measures in obtaining information about which of the following?
    a. Socially unacceptable or private behaviors
    b. Complex research situations when it is difficult to separate processes and interactions
    c. When the researcher is interested in character traits
    d. All of the above

3. Which of the following would be considered disadvantages of using observational data-collection methods?
    a. Individual bias may interfere with the data collection
    b. Ethical concerns may be increasingly significant to researchers using observational data-collection methods
    c. Individual judgments and values influence the perceptions of the observers
    d. All of the above

4. In nursing research, when might questionnaires be used as an appropriate method for data collection?
    a. Whenever expense is a concern for the researcher
    b. When a researcher is interested in obtaining information directly from the subjects
    c. When the researcher needs to collect data from a large group of subjects who are not easily accessible
    d. When accuracy is of the utmost importance to the researcher

5. Which of the following would be considered advantages of using existing records or available data to answer a research question?
    a. The use of available data reduces the risk of researcher bias in data collection
    b. Time involvement in the research study can be reduced by the use of available records or data
    c. Consistent collection of information over periods of time allows the researcher to study trends
    d. All of the above

Activity 6: Web-Based Activity

Go to www.mriresearch.org. The current project of Midwest Research Institute (MRI) is the development of the NDNQI.

1. What do these initials mean?

2. How many quality indicators form the core of NDNQI?

3. Scroll down to "Sample Data Collection Instruments" and click on it. Then click on the "Monthly Patient Fall Report." Into what category of data collection instruments would you place this form?

Activity 7: Evidence-Based Practice Activity

Go to http://www.muhc-ebn.mcgill.ca/. Click on "EBN Guides & Tools" in the list in the middle of the page. Scroll to the "Other Resources" section of the listings. Click on "Practising Evidence-based Nursing." Click on "Sample scenarios, search strategies. . ." Click on "therapy" and read the vignette that comes up. Click on the *JAMA* citation at the end of the vignette. Read the summary of the article that appears.

1. What was the method used in this study? Was it appropriate?

2. If you were a school nurse, would you change your practice based on the evidence provided in this study? Explain your answer.

POST-TEST

Read each question thoroughly and then circle the correct answer.

1. What is the process of translating concepts that are of interest to the researcher into observable and measurable phenomena?
   a. Objectivism
   b. Systematization
   c. Subjectivism
   d. Operationalization

2. Answering research questions pertaining to psychosocial variables can best be answered by using which data-gathering technique(s)?
   a. Observation
   b. Interviews
   c. Questionnaires
   d. All of the above

3. Collection of data from each subject in the same or in a similar manner is known as:
   a. Repetition
   b. Dualism
   c. Consistency
   d. Recidivism

4. Consistency of observations between two or more observers is known as:
   a. Intrarater reliability
   b. Interrater reliability
   c. Consistency reliability
   d. Repetitive reliability

5. Physiological and biological measurement might be used by nurse researchers when studying which of these variables? (Select all that apply.)
   a. A comparison of student nurses' ACT scores and their GPAs
   b. Hypertensive clients' responses to a stress test
   c. Children's dietary patterns
   d. The degree of pain relief achieved following guided imagery

6. Scientific observations should fulfill which of the following conditions?
   a. Observations are consistent with the study objectives.
   b. Observations are standardized and systematically recorded.
   c. Observations are checked and controlled.
   d. All of the above

7. In a research study, a participant observer spent regularly scheduled hours in a homeless shelter and occasionally stayed overnight. The people staying in the home were told that this person was conducting a research study. The researcher freely engaged in conversation and openly observed the homeless. What is the observational role of the researcher?
   a. Concealment without intervention
   b. Concealment with intervention
   c. No concealment without intervention
   d. No concealment with intervention

8. In unstructured observation, which of the following might occur? (Select all that apply.)
   a. Extensive field notes are recorded.
   b. Subjects are informed what behaviors are being observed.
   c. The researcher frequently records interesting anecdotes.
   d. All of the above

9. Which of the following is not consistent with a Likert scale?
   a. It contains close-ended items.
   b. It contains open-ended items.
   c. It contains lists of statements.
   d. Items are evaluated on the amount of agreement.

10. Although it is acceptable to use multiple instruments within a research study, the study is more acceptable if only one method is used for the data collection.
    a. True
    b. False

11. Social desirability is seldom a concern for researchers when the data-collection method used in the study is interviews.
    a. True
    b. False

12. A researcher desires to use a questionnaire in a study but cannot find one that will gather the information desired about a particular variable. The decision is made to develop a new instrument. Which of the following should the researcher do?
    a. Define the construct, formulate the items, and assess the items for content validity
    b. Develop instructions for users and pilot the instrument
    c. Estimate reliability and validity
    d. All of the above

13. The researcher who invests significant amounts of time in the development of an instrument has a professional responsibility to publish the results.
    a. True
    b. False

14. In order to evaluate the adequacy of various data-collection methods, which of the following should be observed in the written research report?
    a. Clear identification of the rationale for selecting a physiological measure
    b. The problems of bias and reactivity are addressed with observational measures
    c. There is a clear explanation of how interviews were conducted and how interviewers were trained
    d. All of the above

15. In conducting a research study, the researcher has a responsibility to ensure that all study subjects received the same information and data was collected from all participants in the same manner.
    a. True
    b. False

Please check with your instructor for the answers to the post-test.

REFERENCES

Davison BJ, Goldenberg SL, Gleave ME, et al. (2003). Provision of individualized information to men and their partners to facilitate treatment decision making in prostate cancer, *Oncol Nurs Forum* 30(1):107-114.

Koniak-Griffin D, Verzemnieks IL, Anderson NLR, et al. (2003). Nurse visitation for adolescent mothers: Two-year infant health and maternal outcomes, *Nurs Res* 52(2):127-136.

McGill University Health Centre Department of Nursing, Nursing Research, Academic Practice and Professional Development: Research & Clinical Resources for Evidence-based Nursing (EBN). Accessed July 21, 2005 from http://www.muhc-ebn.mcgill.ca/.

Midwest Research Institute. Accessed July 21, 2005 from www.mriresearch.org.

Plach SK, Stevens PE, Moss VA (2004) Social role experiences of women living with rheumatoid arthritis, *J Family Nurs* 10(1):33-49.

Van Cleve L, Bossert E, Beecroft P, et al. (2004). The pain experience of children with leukemia during the first year after diagnosis, *Nurs Res* 53(1):1-10.

Reliability and Validity

INTRODUCTION

If someone tells you, "Hey, I found a new restaurant that you will really love," you will consider that information from at least two perspectives before you spend your money there. First, does this person know what she is talking about when it comes to your taste in food? Second, has this person given you good information about food in the past?

You answer "no" to the first question. You prefer seafood served in an elegant setting, and your friend prefers pizza served in a place with sawdust on the floor. Using this information, you will consider her opinion to be invalid for you. You will never give this restaurant another thought.

But if you answer "yes" to the first question because you share similar tastes in food, you will move on to the second question. You remember the tough fettuccini, the superb Southern fried chicken, the unbaked pizza dough, and the hockey-puck biscuits from earlier recommendations. It is likely that while you and your friend share food preferences, her information is not reliable. You can't trust her to give you good information over time. If you are feeling like an adventure, you may try the new restaurant or you may not.

Validity and reliability of the data-collection instruments used in a study are to be regarded in the same way that you would consider your friend's advice about restaurants. Is the instrument valid? Does it provide me with accurate information? Is the instrument reliable? Does it provide me with consistent information whenever it is used? Consideration of both validity and reliability influences your confidence in the results of the study.

LEARNING OUTCOMES

On completion of this chapter, the student should be able to do the following:

- Discuss how measurement error can affect the outcomes of a research study.
- Discuss the purposes of reliability and validity.
- Define reliability.
- Discuss the concepts of stability, equivalence, and homogeneity as they relate to reliability.
- Compare and contrast the estimates of reliability.

- Define validity.
- Compare and contrast content, criterion-related, and construct validity.
- Identify the criteria for critiquing the reliability and validity of measurement tools.
- Use the critiquing criteria to evaluate the reliability and validity of measurement tools.
- Discuss how evidence related to reliability and validity contributes to clinical decision-making.

Activity 1

Either random error (R) or systematic error (S) may occur in a research study. For each of the following examples, identify the type of measurement error and how the error might be corrected.

1. _____ The scale used to obtain daily weights was inaccurate by 3 pounds less than actual weight.

   Correction:

2. _____ Students chose the socially acceptable responses on an instrument to assess attitudes toward AIDS patients.

   Correction:

3. _____ Confusion existed among the evaluators on how to score the wound healing.

   Correction:

4. _____ The subjects were nervous about taking the psychological tests.

   Correction:

Activity 2

Validity is the concern of whether the measurement tools are actually measuring what they are supposed to measure. Use the terms from the following list to complete each of the items in this activity.

Concurrent validity   Content validity   Contrasted groups

Construct validity   Convergent validity   Criterion-related validity

Divergent validity   Face validity   Factor analysis

Hypothesis testing   Multitrait-multimethod   Predictive validity
                             approach

Rating from a panel
of experts

1. "_____ was supported by factor analysis yielding the three sub-scales of communication, consistent use, and correct use self efficacy. In addition, _____ was supported in that subscales allowed investigators to differ-entiate between regular and irregular condom users. Cronbach's alpha coefficient rated between .72 and .78 for the subscales, and was .85 for the total scale." (Thato et al. 2005)

2. _____ is an intuitive, preliminary type of instrument evaluation.

3. "In studies using [the descriptive phenomenological] method, the researcher develops a "rationale for investigating an experience and for seeking certain types of data in particu-lar settings and circumstances" (Porter, 1998, p. 22). Data to be included were the mothers' perceptions, actions, and intentions relevant to helping the young adult with [traumatic brain injury], and the interview guide was developed accordingly. Favorable views of its _____ were provided by an eligible mother who did not participate and by the case manager who worked with eligible mothers." (Wongvatunyu & Porter 2005)

4. "The survey design process began with the school nurses who told the authors and under-graduate nursing students what information they sought from the survey. The authors and nine undergraduate community health nursing students used these ideas to develop a one-page questionnaire entitled "Breakfast Survey." The school nurses and nutritionist (n = 3) served as _____. They reviewed and revised the survey before it was sent to the school principal for final approval." (Sweeney & Horishita 2005)

5. "Previous studies have demonstrated that the Daily Hassles for Adolescents Inventory has good _____, as evidenced by its significant relationship to adjustment measures." (Guthrie et al. 2002)

6. Construct validity, an assessment of the relationship between the instrument and the underlying theory, can be measured in several ways. List three of these: _____, _____, and _____.

7. "A 2-week test-retest of 108 of the original 599 [participants] yielded an alpha of .94. Five judges with expertise in the area of the code for nurses examined the instrument for _____. Validity of each item required agreement among four of the five experts." (Martin et al. 2003)

Activity 3

An instrument is considered reliable if it is accurate and consistent. If the concept being studied is stable, the same results should occur when measurement is repeated.

1. Three concepts related to reliability include _____, _____, and _____.

2. Give an example of each of the two types of tests for stability.

3. In what instance would it be better to use an alternate form rather than a test-retest measure for stability?

4. Homogeneity is a measure of internal consistency. All items on the instrument should be complementary and measure the same characteristic or concepts. For each of the following examples, identify which of the following tests for homogeneity is described:

    (1) Item-total correlations
    (2) Split-half reliability
    (3) Kuder-Richardson (KR-20) coefficient
    (4) Cronbach's alpha

    a. _____   The odd items of the test had a high correlation with the even numbers of the test.

    b. _____   Each item on the test using a 5-point Likert scale had a moderate correlation with every other item on the test.

    c. _____   Each item on the test ranged in correlation from 0.62 to 0.89 with the total.

    d. _____   Each item on the true-false test had a moderate correlation with every other item on the test.

5. Review the information about the instruments used in the Davison et al. study in Appendix D of the text; e.g., the Patient Information Program, the Control Preferences Scale, the survey questionnaire, the Spielberger State Anxiety Inventory, and the Center for Epidemiologic Studies Depression Scale.

    a. Think about the concept of face validity. Think about the variables being addressed in the study. Would you conclude that these instruments had face validity for this study?

b. What information is given to the reader about the Center for Epidemiologic Studies Depression Scale?

c. How does this information influence your level of confidence in the results of this study?

Activity 4: Web-Based Activity

Go to www.cdc.gov. Click on "A-Z Index" (at the top of the page). Click on "H," then on "Health-Related Quality of Life," then on "Methods and Measures." Scroll to "Measurement Properties" and click. Scroll to the Nelson, Holtzman, Bolen, Stanwyck, and Mack article, and click on it. Read the first part of the article. What measures of health-related quality of life are considered to have high reliability and high validity?

Activity 5

In this activity you will use the critiquing criteria listed in chapter 15 of the text to think about the Van Cleve et al. study in Appendix B of the text.

1. How many instruments for data collection were used in this study?

2. Read the validity and reliability information provided for each instrument and answer the critiquing questions in chapter 15. Complete the table below using "Y" for yes, "N" for no, and "?" if you don't know or can't find the answer.

CRITIQUING QUESTIONS

Instrument	#1	#2	#3	#4	#5	#6	#7	#8
Poker Chip								
Preschool Body Outline								
Adolescent Pediatric Pain								
Dot Matrix								
Pediatric Pain Coping								
Perception of Management Effectiveness								
Functional Status								

☀ Activity 6: Evidence-Based Practice Activity

Now think about the study reviewed in Activity 5. Look at the table you have completed regarding the reliability and validity measures of the instruments used in the study. Assume you are a nurse in pediatric oncology. How would you use the results of this study to guide your practice?

POST-TEST

Using the following terms, complete the sentences for the type of validity or reliability discussed. Terms may be used more than once.

Content	Test-retest
Factor analysis	Cronbach's alpha
Convergent	Alternate or parallel form
Divergent	Interrater
Concurrent	

1. In tests for reliability, the self-efficacy scale had a(n) _____ of 0.88, demonstrating internal consistency for the new measure.

2. The ABC social support scale demonstrated _____ validity with correlation of 0.84 with the XYZ interpersonal relationships scale.

3. _____ validity was supported with a correlation of 0.42 between the ABC social support scale and the QRS loneliness scale.

4. The investigator established _____ validity through evaluation of the cardiac recovery scale by a panel of cardiac clinical nurse specialists. All items were rated 0 to 5 for importance to recovery and only items scoring above an average of 3 were kept in the final scale.

5. The results of the _____ were that all the items clustered around three factors, lending support to the notion that there are three dimensions of coping.

6. The observations were rated by three experts. The _____ reliability among the observers was 94%.

7. To assess _____ reliability, subjects completed the locus of control questionnaire at the beginning of the project and 2 weeks later. The correlation of 0.86 supports the stability of the concept.

8. Bennett et al. (1996) developed an instrument called the Cardiac Event Threat Questionnaire (CTQ). They established _____ validity by reviewing the literature reviewing concerns identified by patients recovering from a cardiac event, and had the items critiqued by a panel of experts.

9. The results of the CTQ that measured threat were highly correlated with the results of a test measuring negative emotions. This established _____ validity.

10. Bennett et al. (1996) reported that internal consistency reliabilities of the five factors of the CTQ were computed with the _____ statistic.

Please check with your instructor for the answers to the post-test.

REFERENCES

Bennett SJ et al. (1996). Development of an instrument to measure threat related to cardiac events, *Nurs Res* 45:266-270.

Davison BJ, Goldenberg SL, Gleave ME, et al. (2003). Provision of individualized information to men and their partners to facilitate treatment decision making in prostate cancer, *Oncol Nurs Forum* 30(1):107-114.

Guthrie BJ, Young AM, Williams DR, et al. (2002). African-American girls' smoking habits and day-to-day experience with racial discrimination, *Nurs Res* 53(3):183-190.

Martin P, Yarbrough S, Alfred D (2003). Professional values held by baccalaureate and associate degree nursing students, *J Nurs Scholarsh*, 35(3):291-296.

Nelson DE, Holtzman D, Bolen J, et al. (2001). Reliability and validity of measures from the Behavioral Risk Factor Surveillance System (BRFSS) *Sozial- und Praventiv Medizin* 1:(46 Suppl) S3–42.

Sweeney NM, Horishita N (2005). The breakfast-eating habits of inner city high school students, *J Sch Nurs*, 21(2):100-105.

Thato S, Hanna KM, Rodcumdee B (2005). Translation and validation of the condom self-efficacy scale with Thai adolescents and young adults, *J Nurs Scholarsh*, 37(1):36-40.

U.S. Department of Health and Human Services: Centers for Disease Control. Accessed July 21, 2005 from http://www.cdc.gov/.

Van Cleve L, Bossert E, Beecroft P, et al. (2004). The pain experience of children with leukemia during the first year after diagnosis, *Nurs Res* 53(1):1-10.

Wongvatunyu S, Porter EJ (2005). Mothers' experience of helping young adults with traumatic brain injury, *J Nurs Scholarsh*, 37(1):48-56.

Data Analysis: Descriptive and Inferential Statistics

INTRODUCTION

Measurement is critical to any study. The practitioner is interested in the similarity between the measurements used in a study and those usually found in his or her practice. The researcher thinks about how to measure relevant variables while reading the literature and thinking through the theoretical rationale for the study. Both the practitioner and the researcher wonder about how much faith they can put in the measurements reported.

Practitioners and researchers know that the perfect set of measurements does not exist. The researcher's task is to clearly define the variables, choose accurate measurement tools, and clearly explain how the statistical tools were used. Your task as a practitioner who critically reads research is to consider the researcher's explanation of how and why specific descriptive and inferential statistics were used and ask, "What do these numbers tell me?"

Descriptive statistics are valuable for summarizing data and allowing us to look at salient features about a group of data, but practitioners usually want more information. They want to be able to read about an intervention used with a specific group of individuals and consider the usefulness of that intervention with the clients in their care. The use of inferential statistics provides a way for practitioners to look at the data in a study and decide how easily the results can be generalized to the clients they see on a daily basis.

Initially, numbers tend to be intimidating. The best way to eliminate this source of intimidation is to jump in and play with the numbers. Keep reminding yourself that you have the intelligence and skills to do this. Use the mantras of "I think I can. I think I can." (*The Little Engine that Could)* and "practice, practice, practice," and you will have data analysis mastered. Also keep in mind that this is a life-long learning process. There are still times when you will read a study with a new twist to the use of a statistical procedure, and back you'll go to the reference books, or pick up the phone to call a colleague.

This chapter is designed to help you with the skills part of the task. First, the exercises in this chapter will provide you with some practice in working with the concept of measurement. Second, you will have the opportunity to think through some of the decisions relevant to the use of descriptive and inferential statistics. The bulk of your effort will be spent digesting data from the studies included in the text.

LEARNING OUTCOMES

On completion of this chapter, the student should be able to do the following:

- Differentiate between descriptive and inferential statistics.
- State the purposes of descriptive statistics.
- Identify the levels of measurement in a research study.
- Describe a frequency distribution.
- List measures of central tendency and their use.
- List measures of variability and their use.
- Identify the purpose of inferential statistics.
- Distinguish between a parameter and a statistic.
- Explain the concept of probability as it applies to the analysis of sample data.
- Distinguish between type I and type II error and its effect on a study's outcome.
- Distinguish between parametric and nonparametric tests.
- List the commonly used statistical tests and their purposes.
- Critically analyze the statistics used in published research studies.

Activity 1

Before you start any of the activities for chapter 16, make life easier for yourself—create tools that will provide a shortcut. Create a set of reference cards that can also serve as flash cards.

Create your own set of "statistical assistants." Once the cards are finished, carry them with you to the library, or set them on the desk while working on the Internet. Use them when reading research reports. Before long, you will be able to read a piece of research without referring to the stack of statistical assistants, and you will master the best shortcut of all: memorizing the statistical notation. Flipping through the pages of a book looking for a statistical symbol before you can evaluate the use of the statistic will no longer be required.

Gather the following supplies: package of 3 x 5 index cards, preferably lined on one side; 6 pens or a combination of pens and highlighters with 6 different colors; 1 broad-tipped, black-ink marker.

1. Make two key cards first. On one of the 3 x 5 cards, on the side without lines, use the broad-tipped, black marker and write "NAME OF INFERENTIAL STATISTICAL TECHNIQUE." Take the second 3 x 5 card and write "NAME OF DESCRIPTIVE TECHNIQUE" on the unlined side.

2. Turn the *inferential statistics* card over to the lined side. With one of the colored pens, write "Symbol" on the first line. Complete this side of the card with five more categories of information using a different line and a different-colored pen for each line for each category. An example of the lined side of the card follows:

Symbol

# of independent variables (IV)

IV's level of measurement

HR = relationship? (# of variables?)

Parametric/nonparametric?

# of dependent variables (DV)

DV's level of measurement

differences? (# of groups?)

3. Do the same with the *descriptive statistics* card. An example follows:

Symbol

Central tendency

Variability

Frequency

4. Each line of the key card should be in a different color. Next, create a stack of statistical assistants.

5. Take a blank card. On the front of each card (unlined side) write the full name of one of the statistical tools using the broad-tipped, black marker (or whatever marker was used to write on the front of the key card) (Example: *Pearson product moment correlation*).

6. Turn the card over and write the information that corresponds to the appropriate category on the key card on the appropriate line using the appropriate color. If assistance with choosing the appropriate information to put on each line is needed, refer to Table 16-1 and the Critical Thinking Decision Pathways in chapter 16 of the text. For example, the lined side of the Pearson product moment correlation would read as follows:

r

IV = 1

DV = 1

IV = at least interval

DV = at least interval

relationship (2 variables)

parametric

7. These cards will fit into an envelope or any of the small plastic cases that can be purchased from the local bookstore. They will slip into a book bag, briefcase, or backpack with ease.

Activity 2

Match the level of measurement found in Column B with the appropriate example(s) in Column A. The levels of measurement in Column B will be used more than once. Table 16-1 from the text can assist you.

Column A

1. _____ Amount of emesis

2. _____ Scores on the ACT, SAT, or the GRE

3. _____ Height or weight

4. _____ High, moderate, low level of social support

5. _____ Satisfaction with nursing care

6. _____ Use or nonuse of contraception

7. _____ Amount of empathy

8. _____ Number of feet or meters walked

9. _____ Type A or Type B behavior

10. _____ Body temperature measured with centigrade thermometer

Column B

a. Nominal
b. Ordinal
c. Interval
d. Ratio

Activity 3

If you have taken a course in statistics, you are familiar with the statistical notation used to refer to specific types of descriptive statistics. This activity will serve as a quick review. If you have not yet taken a statistics course, this exercise will provide you with enough information to recognize some of the statistical notations.

This is a *reverse* crossword puzzle; therefore, the puzzle is already completed. Your task is to identify the appropriate clue for each answer found in the puzzle. List the correct clue answers in the spaces provided following the puzzle and clues.

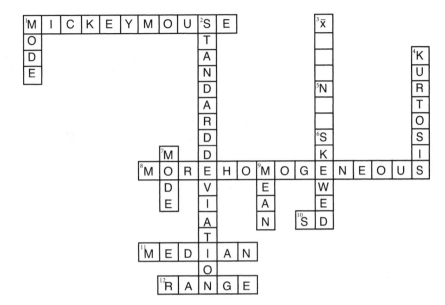

The Clues

a. Measure of central tendency used with interval or ratio data
b. Abbreviation for the number of measures in a given data set (the measures may be individual people or some smaller piece of data like blood pressure readings)
c. Measure of variation that shows the lowest and highest number in a set
d. Can describe the height of a distribution
e. Old abbreviation for the mean
f. Marks the "score" where 50% of the scores are higher and 50% are lower
g. Describes a distribution characterized by a tail
h. Abbreviation for standard deviation
i. 68% of the values in a normal distribution fall between ± 1 of this statistic
j. Goofy's best friend
k. Very unstable
l. The values that occur most frequently in a data set
m. Describes a set of data with a standard deviation of 3 when compared to a set of data with a standard deviation of 12

Across	Down
1.	1.
3.	2.
5.	4.
8.	6.
10.	7.
11.	9.
12.	

Activity 4

Read the following excerpts from specific studies. Identify both the independent and dependent variable(s) and indicate what level of measurement would apply. You may find the Critical Thinking Decision Path in the textbook to be very helpful in answering these questions.

1. "Because BMI in children is gender and age specific, the Centers for Disease Control and Prevention (CDC, 2004) recommends that BMI be categorized by percentile as underweight (<5%), normal weight (between 5% and 85%), at risk for overweight (between 85% and 95%), and overweight (>95%).

    Among the students assessed, 21% met the CDC criteria for overweight, and 17% were at risk for overweight. Thus, 38% were at an increased risk for obesity-related illnesses in the future (Table 3)." (Gance-Cleveland & Bushmiaer, 2005, p. 68)

    a. Name the variable of interest.

    b. Identify the level of measurement of this variable.

2. "At 4 months, the mean weight change in the [educational] intervention group was .81 lbs., while the mean weight change in the standard care group was 7.17 lbs." (Littrell et al., 2003, p. 240)

    a. Name the independent variable(s).

    b. Name the dependent variable(s).

    c. Identify the level of measurement of each variable.

3. "Only two of the IVs contributed significantly to prediction of postpartum women's health: postpartum stress scores ($sr^2 = .07$) and depression scores ($sr^2 = .14$). The three combined IVs contributed another .22 in shared variability. Altogether, 43% (42% adjusted) of the variability in postpartum women's health status was explained by these three IVs." (Hung, 2004, p. 348)

    a. Name the independent variable(s).

    b. Name the dependent variable(s).

Activity 5

Use the list of terms to complete the items in this activity. Some terms may be used more than once.

ANOVA	Correlation	Nonparametric statistics
Null hypothesis	Parameter	Parametric statistics
Practical significance	Probability	Research hypothesis
Sampling error	Statistic	Statistical significance
Type I error	Type II error	

1. The _____ states that there is no difference between the groups in the study or no association between the variables under study. Its usefulness to a study is that it is the only relationship that can be tested through the use of statistical tools.

2. _____ is an example of the use of _____.

3. It is impossible to prove that the _____ is true.

4. The tendency for statistics to fluctuate from one sample to another is known as the _____.

5. The term _____ refers to a characteristic of the population while the term _____ refers to a characteristic of a sample drawn from a population.

6. When investigators are studying the association between variables, they often will use statistics that measure _____.

7. _____ occurs when the investigator does not find statistical significance but a real difference exists in the world. A _____ occurs when the investigator concludes that there is a real (statistically significant) difference but, in reality, there is no difference.

8. The relative frequency of an event in repeated trials under similar conditions is known as _____ and provides the theoretical basis for inferential statistics.

9. A statistically significant finding based on a change of 3 mm Hg in systolic blood pressure in a sample of healthy individuals likely would have little _____.

10. _____ refer to those tools used when data are collected at the ordinal or nominal level of measurement.

11. When a finding is tested and found to be unlikely to have happened by chance, the investigators report _____ for that particular finding.

12. When a probability level is calculated as $p < 0.05$ and the investigator had set the alpha level of significance at 0.05, the investigator must reject the _____ and accept the _____.

13. Identify the components of the following statistical test result: X2 (6, n=213) = 33.0, p < .0001. Match the component with its correct name.

_____ X2   a.   Sample size

_____ 6   b.   Degrees of freedom

_____ n = 213   c.   Chi-square symbol

_____ 33.0   d.   Probability level

_____ p < .0001   e.   Chi-square test statistic

Activity 6

Practice using the cards. The data in this table contains information from a study. Use the statistical assistant cards you developed in Activity 1 to answer the questions that follow the table.

Table 4. Relationship of Postpartum Health to Demographic and Perinatal Variables

Variables	n	Postpartum Health* M + SD	Test	df	p
This childbirth experience			t = -3.38	859	.01
Satisfying	784	2.09 ± 1.98			
Unsatisfying	77	2.89 ± 2.16			
Preferred sex of this baby			t = 2.14	660	.03
Had gender preference	345	2.35 ± 2.18			
Didn't matter	516	2.04 ± 1.87			

(Hung, 2004, p. 349)
*Scores on instrument used to measure postpartum health with higher score indicating poorer health status.

1.   In your own words, explain what it is the researcher wants you to learn from Table 4.

2.   What descriptive statistics are present in Table 4?

3.   What inferential statistic was used with these data?

4. Name the independent variable(s) and the dependent variable(s).

5. What is the level of measurement for each of the variables listed in item #4?

6. State the null hypothesis(es) in this study.

Activity 7

Using the studies in Appendices A through D in the textbook, answer the following questions regarding the use of descriptive and inferential statistics in each study. Once again, use the Critical Thinking Decision Path in chapter 16 of the textbook.

1. Were descriptive statistics used in the study?

   a. Koniak-Griffin et al.

   b. Van Cleve et al.

   c. Plach et al.

   d. Davison et al.

2. What data were summarized and/or explained through the use of descriptive statistics?

   a. Koniak-Griffin et al.

   b. Van Cleve et al.

   c. Plach et al.

   d. Davison et al.

3. Were the descriptive statistics used appropriately?

   a. Koniak-Griffin et al.

   b. Van Cleve et al.

   c. Plach et al.

   d. Davison et al.

4. Did any of the four studies rely more heavily on the use of descriptive statistics than the others? If so, why do you think this occurred?

5. Now turn to the inferential statistics. Which of the four studies in the appendices used some type of inferential statistic to manage the data?
   a. Koniak-Griffin et al.
   b. Van Cleve et al.
   c. Plach et al.
   d. Davison et al.

6. Name the inferential statistical tools used in the studies and the variables used with each inferential tool.

   a. Koniak-Griffin et al.

   b. Van Cleve et al.

   c. Plach et al.

   d. Davison et al.

7. For which study was the data analysis the easiest to read? Can you figure out why the one you named was the easiest to read?

Activity 8: Web-Based Activity

1. Go to http://www.yahooligans.yahoo.com and click on "Science and Nature." Then click on "Animals@" and then "Endangered Species." Find the link to "ES2000 Endangered Species of the Next Millennium" and click on it. Click on "English version" and click on "Facts" in the Facts and Quotes area. Read the paragraph about the blue whale. What descriptive information did you find in this paragraph?

2. Now go the http://www.cdc.gov and click on "Injury and Violence" in the Health and Safety Topics found on the left-hand side of the webpage. Click on the Intimate Partner Violence site. Scroll down and skim the contents of this site.
   - What percent of the women murdered by their intimate partner had visited an emergency department within two years of the homicide?
   - What percent of these women had had at least one injury visit to an emergency department?

Activity 9: Evidence-Based Practice Activity

Evidence-based practice means that you base practice decisions on the best evidence available. In the ideal world, this means practitioners would have a stack of experimental studies with clear conclusions that have direct relevance to an immediate clinical concern. Obviously, this is seldom the case. We use our brains and the best practice information available, and intervene and evaluate.

Assume that the CDC statistics from Activity 8 about intimate partner violence (IPV) have been consistently reported across several studies of varying designs and sample sizes. What, if any, implications would exist for RNs working in an emergency department?

POST-TEST

1. Two outpatient clinics measured client waiting time as one indicator of effectiveness. The mean and standard deviation of waiting time in minutes is reported below. Which outpatient clinic would you prefer, assuming that all other things are equal? Explain your answer.

	Clinic 1	Clinic 2
Mean (in minutes)	40	25
Standard deviation (in minutes)	10	45

2. You are responsible for ordering a new supply of hospital gowns for your unit. Which measure of central tendency would be the most useful in your decision-making? Explain your answer.

3. Use the table below to answer the questions that follow. Responses to each of the items was either True or False, with True scored as a 1 and False scored as 0.

Table 1: Means and Standard Deviations on Survey Questions (N = 116)

	M	**SD**
Every Saturday night, a girl in your class has a party. She invites all your friends but never invites you. You are a victim of bullying.	.17	.38
One Friday you wear a new dress to school, and your best friend tells you on the way to class that it makes you look fat. She is bullying you.	.67	.47
A girl in your class regularly starts rumors about people at school that are true. This girl is a bully.	.86	.35
A group of girls is passing notes in class, and when certain people raise their hands, all of the girls giggle. These girls are bullies.	.62	.49
When girls tease each other, it can have lasting effects on self-esteem and body image.	.95	.22
Bullies exist at my school.	.92	.27

(Raskauskas & Stoltz, 2004, p. 211)

   a. About which statement was there the widest range of responses? What statistic did you use to answer this question?

   b. About which statements did the respondents (adolescent girls) have the most agreement? Explain your answer.

   c. The second item of the five items listed was considered to be benign, (i.e., was not a bullying incident). How would you interpret the mean and standard deviation associated with this item?

Please check with your instructor for the answers to the post-test.

REFERENCES

Davison BJ, Goldenberg SL, Gleave ME, et al. (2003). Provision of individualized information to men and their partners to facilitate treatment decision making in prostate cancer, *Oncol Nurs Forum* 30(1):107-114.

Gance-Cleveland B, Bushmiaer M (2005). Arkansas school nurses' role in statewide assessment of body mass index to screen for overweight children and adolescents, *J Sch Nurs* 21(2): 64-69.

Hung CH (2004). Predictors of postpartum women's health status, *J Nurs Scholarsh.* 36(4): 345-351.

Koniak-Griffin D, Verzemnieks IL, Anderson NLR, et al. (2003). Nurse visitation for adolescent mothers: Two-year infant health and maternal outcomes, *Nurs Res* 52(2):127-136.

Littrell KH, Hilligoss NM, Kirshner CD, et al. (2003). The effects of an educational intervention on antipsychotic-induced weight gain, *J Nurs Scholarsh* 35(3):237-241.

Plach SK, Stevens PE, Moss VA (2004) Social role experiences of women living with rheumatoid arthritis, *J Family Nurs* 10(1):33-49.

Raskauskas J, Stoltz AD (2004). Identifying and intervening in relational aggression, *J Sch Nurs* 20(4):209-215.

U.S. Department of Health and Human Services: Centers for Disease Control. Accessed July 22, 2005 from http://www.cdc.gov.

Van Cleve L, Bossert E, Beecroft P, et al. (2004). The pain experience of children with leukemia during the first year after diagnosis, *Nurs Res* 53(1):1-10.

Yahooligans! Accessed July 22, 2005 from http://www.yahooligans.yahoo.com.

Analysis of Findings

INTRODUCTION

As the last sections of a research report, the results and conclusions sections answer the question "So what?" In other words, it is in these two sections that the investigator "makes sense" of the research, critically synthesizes the data, ties them to a theoretical framework, and builds on a body of knowledge. These two sections are a very important part of the research report because they describe the generalizability of the findings and offer recommendations for further research. Well-written, clear, and concise results and conclusions sections provide valuable information for nursing practice. Conversely, poorly written results and conclusions sections will leave a reader bewildered, confused, and wondering how or if the findings are relevant to nursing.

LEARNING OUTCOMES

On completion of this chapter, the student should be able to do the following:

- Discuss the difference between the "Results" section of a study and the "Discussion of the Results" section.
- Identify the format of the "Results" section.
- Determine if both statistically supported and statistically unsupported findings are discussed.
- Determine whether the results are objectively reported.
- Describe how tables and figures are used in a research report.
- List the criteria of a meaningful table.
- Identify the format and components of the "Discussion of the Results" section.
- Determine the purpose of the "Discussion" section.
- Discuss the importance of including generalizations and limitations of a study in the report.
- Determine the purpose of including recommendations in the study report.
- Discuss how the strength, quality, and consistency of evidence provided by the findings are related to a study's limitations, generalizability, and applicability to practice.

Activity 1

Knowing what information to look for and where to find it in the "Results and Discussions" sections of a research report will enable you to interpret the research findings and critique research reports.

Identify the section in which the following information from the research report may be found. Put an **R** in the blank space if the information would be found in the "Results" section and a **D** if the information would be found in the "Discussion" section.

1. _____   Tables/figures

2. _____   Limitations of the study

3. _____   Data analysis related to the literature review

4. _____   Inferences or generalization of results

5. _____   Statistical support or non-support of hypotheses

6. _____   Findings of the hypothesis testing

7. _____   Information about the statistical tests used to analyze hypotheses

8. _____   Application of meaning (makes sense) of data analysis

9. _____   Suggestions for further research

10. _____   Recommendations for nursing practice

Activity 2

Tables are an important part of the data analysis component of a study. This activity will focus on tables.

Read the following paragraph from the Sweeney & Horishita (2005) study on breakfast eating habits. Then review the data in Table 1 from the same study (on the next page). Answer the questions that follow the table.

> Milk consumption decreased as grade level increased, whereas drinking orange juice varied. Cereal-eating varied without pattern, other than to note that 10th-graders had the lowest rate of cereal consumption. Using the chi-square test, no statistically significant associations were found between gender or grade level and the consumption of milk, juice, or cereal. (Sweeney and Horishita, p. 103)

Table 1: Breakfast Eating Habits by Gender and Grade (N = 846)

Variable	Girl % (n)	Boy % (n)	9th % (n)	10th % (n)	11th % (n)	12th % (n)	Total % (n)
Skipped breakfast	61 (258)	54 (214)	53 (163)	65 (168)	56 (81)	54 (70)	57 (486)
Where eat breakfast							
Home	44 (186)	52 (206)	51 (156)	44 (114)	47 (68)	47 (61)	48 (403)
School	12 (49)	15 (60)	15 (46)	11 (29)	16 (23)	12 (16)	14 (115)
Both	3 (12)	3 (13)	2 (7)	4 (10)	5 (7)	0.8 (1)	3 (25)
No answer	41 (174)	30 (120)	32 (96)	41 (106)	33 (48)	40 (51)	36 (303)
When eat breakfast, what consumed							
Milk	30 (126)	32 (129)	35 (107)	31 (80)	27 (40)	26 (33)	31 (261)
Cereal	29 (121)	31 (123)	31 (93)	28 (72)	30 (43)	31 (40)	30 (252)
Orange juice	31 (131)	26 (102)	28 (86)	29 (76)	32 (46)	23 (30)	28 (239)

(Sweeney & Horishita, p. 103)

1. Does the information in the table meet the criteria for a table as described in chapter 17 of the textbook? Explain.

2. Which food was most likely to be eaten for breakfast?

3. Did boys or girls drink the most orange juice?

4. Who declined to answer the most often?

Activity 3

Collect demographic data on the people in your research class. You can decide what data you want to collect but common variables would be age, gender, eye color, hair color (current or underlying), etc. Once the data have been collected, work in groups of no less than 3 but no more than five and create a table that displays these data. Exchange tables with another group. Critique each other's table with the intent of improving the table.

Criteria to consider:
   a. Are data summaries included and not all of the raw data?
   b. Is the title clear? Do you know what data are being presented without needing to read the text?
   c. Are the columns and rows appropriately labeled?
   d. Are there other criteria you want to include? Does your instructor have suggestions?

Activity 4

This activity will give you some practice in the interpretation of research articles. Read the Davison et al. (2003) article in Appendix D of the textbook and answer the following items.

1. The following items pertain to Table 1 of the article.

    a. What is the meaning of the "(N = 74)" on this table?

    b. In which group was the age most variable?

    c. What data did you use to answer item b?

2. Look at Table 3.

    a. What happened to all anxiety and depression scores between the first time and the second time they were measured?

    b. Were any depression scores considered to be clinically relevant?

Now read the study by Koniak-Griffin et al. (2003) in Appendix A of the textbook, and answer the following items.

3. How many individuals are represented by the numbers in Table 1?

4. How many statistically significant findings are reported in Table 2?

Activity 5: Web-Based Activity

1. Go to www.google.com and type "analysis" in the search box. Scroll down and look at the number of the websites that use "analysis" in their description. Look through a few pages (usually 10 sites on each page). On a scale of 1 to 10 (with 1 indicating very little value) indicate where would you place the value of using the word "analysis" as a search term when looking for studies relevant to nursing. Play with modifiers of "analysis" and see if you can get some useful information from this search.

2. Now enter "analysis research studies, nursing" in the search box. How many hits did you get? Skim through the first five pages of listed items. What words seem to be driving the search?

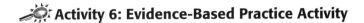## Activity 6: Evidence-Based Practice Activity

Evidence-based practice asks the practitioner to use the "best" evidence available when deciding which interventions to use. The results and discussion section of any study can help you, the practitioner, decide if the study is one that needs to be included in your considerations.

Go to http://evidence.ahc.umn.edu/ebn.htm and click on "Research-based nursing journals." How many journals are listed? How many of these journals have you consulted? Check the library at your school. How many of the journals could you access?

POST-TEST

1. When a research hypothesis is supported through testing, it may be assumed that the hypothesis was which of the following?
   a. Proved
   b. Accepted
   c. Rejected
   d. Disconfirmed

2. Limitations of a study describe its weaknesses.

   True   False

3. The "Results" section of a research study includes all the following **except**:
   a. Hypothesis testing results
   b. Tables and figures
   c. Statistical test description
   d. Limitations of the study

4. Unsupported hypotheses mean that the study is of little value in improving practice.

   True   False

5. Tables in research reports should meet all of the following criteria **except**:
   a. Clear and concise
   b. Restate the text narrative
   c. Economize the text
   d. Supplement the text narrative

6. The "Discussion" section provides opportunity for the investigator to do all of the following **except**:
   a. Describe implications from the research results
   b. Relate the results to the literature review
   c. Make generalizations to large populations of subjects
   d. Suggest areas for further research

7. Hypothesis testing is described in the "Discussion" section of the research report.

True   False

Please check with your instructor for the answers to the post-test.

REFERENCES

Davison BJ, Goldenberg SL, Gleave ME, et al. (2003). Provision of individualized information to men and their partners to facilitate treatment decision making in prostate cancer, *Oncol Nurs Forum* 30(1):107-114.

Koniak-Griffin D, Verzemnieks IL, Anderson NLR, et al. (2003). Nurse visitation for adolescent mothers: Two-year infant health and maternal outcomes, *Nurs Res* 52(2):127-136.

Sweeney NM, Horishita N (2005). The breakfast-eating habits of inner city high school students, *J Sch Nurs* 21(2):100-105.

University of Minnesota. "Evidence-Based Health Care Project." Accessed July 21, 2005 from http://evidence.ahc.umn.edu/ebn.htm.

Evaluating Quantitative Research

INTRODUCTION

Chapter 18 in the textbook includes two thorough critiques of quantitative studies. Heerman and Craft (the authors) addressed the various critiquing criteria that have been presented in all previous chapters. They have very carefully walked you through each item. The result is a complete critique of two separate studies.

Both of these critiques reflect the level of analysis desired for an article that the RN had decided was relevant to practice. If you want to produce a critique at this level of thoroughness, it will take time. It would not be uncommon for a novice reader of research to use two to three hours (maybe more) to complete such a critique. Usually novice readers of research find the task tedious and, not infrequently, difficult. The more often you read and critique studies in this manner, the easier (and more interesting) reading research becomes. The easier it becomes, the more quickly you can complete a critique. To get started, you just have to pick a place, dive in, and do it.

One way of getting started is to work on a weekly schedule to master this skill. Each week, find one research article relevant to your favorite area of nursing and critique that article using the steps outlined in the textbook. At the end of one year, you will have read four dozen studies (take time off for holidays, your birthday, and one "I just forgot"). By this time, you will have mastered research critiques.

As mentioned earlier, this level of reading and critiquing is most often used when you have a reasonable expectation that a specific study will be useful in your professional practice. But not all relevant articles will be found in the journals that are devoted specifically to your area of clinical expertise. You must search several journals to find all of the articles that can be useful. When you do find an article that appears to be practice-relevant, you need to assess the article quickly so you can decide whether it requires more in-depth analysis.

LEARNING OUTCOMES

On completion of this chapter, the student should be able to do the following:

- Identify the purpose of the critiquing process.
- Describe the criteria for each step of the critiquing process.
- Evaluate the strengths or weaknesses of a research report.
- Apply levels of evidence to evaluation of a quantitative research report.
- Discuss the implications of the findings of a research report for evidence-based nursing practice.
- Construct a critique of a research report.

Activity 1

This quick reading of articles demands that you, the reader, consider the same aspects of a study that you would consider if completing a more detailed critique but in a more superficial manner. This type of reading is called "inspectional reading" (Adler & Van Doren 1972). Mastering inspectional reading is essential, but is frequently overlooked in regard to analytical skills. Frequently, professional reading must be squeezed into a small window of available time. Improving your quick reading skills will help you to sort through the reading that is required to maintain and expand your knowledge base.

But what is this inspectional reading? It is the second level in a set of skills described by Adler and Van Doren (1972). The first skill is elementary reading, which is usually accomplished by the time you have completed the fourth grade. Level two is inspectional reading. Level three is analytical reading where the reader is trying very hard to understand what the author is attempting to share, and is the level of reading required to produce a critique of a research study. Level four is syntopical reading, which requires intense effort to synthesize ideas from many sources.

Inspectional reading has two components. The first is called "systematic skimming" and the second is called "superficial reading."

Systematic skimming is the first thing anyone should do when approaching a reading assignment. It requires only a few minutes to skim an article (it may take up to an hour if you are skimming a complete book). Let's assume that you are going to skim a hard copy of a research article.

- Read the title and the abstract.
- Read the biographical information about the authors/researchers.
- Pay close attention to the clinical area and the population of subjects.
- Read the conclusions section.
- Ask yourself "Are the individuals in this study comparable to the people in which I am interested? Is the problem/clinical area/question close to my interests?" If you answer "no" to these questions, put this study down and go to the next one. If you answer "yes" to either of these questions, then proceed to superficial reading of the article.

If you are undecided about whether it is related to your clinical concerns, proceed to superficial reading of the article.

Superficial reading requires that you read the article from beginning to end without stopping. Do not take notes. Do not highlight. (Hide your highlighter so you won't even be tempted.) Do not use the dictionary to understand words that you don't know. Do not stop and think "I wonder what they meant by that." Just read!

When you have completed the article, take a deep breath and ask yourself these questions.

- What do I remember about the study? The question? The methods? The results? The discussion?
- Was this clinical or basic research?
- Was it experimental, nonexperimental, or qualitative?
- Where would I put it on the level of evidence scale?
- Did anything in the study raise any ethical questions? (Listen to yourself. If there is even a twinge of a question, listen to yourself.)
- Does it fit my interests? (If the answer is "no," move on to the next article. If the answer is "maybe," put it in a come-back-to-later stack. If the answer is "yes," then proceed to more detailed reading and perhaps jot down the notes that would be necessary to complete a critique.)

Now let's practice. There is one activity for this chapter. The Koniak-Griffin et al. article (Appendix A of the textbook) has been used for several activities throughout this study guide. However, it is possible that you have not read it completely from beginning to end. **Do so now.** Read the Koniak-Griffin et al. article using the inspectional reading strategies. When you have completed reading the article, answer the questions related to inspectional reading. Make a decision: Is this an article that would assist you in building the evidence base for the area of nursing that most appeals to you?

When you have completed your reading, turn to the answers in the back of the study guide.

Note: There is no post-test for this chapter. Enjoy the break!

REFERENCES

Adler MJ, Van Doren C (1972). *How to Read a Book*. New York: Simon & Schuster.
Koniak-Griffin D, Verzemnieks IL, Anderson NLR, et al. (2003). Nurse visitation for adolescent mothers: Two-year infant health and maternal outcomes, *Nurs Res* 52(2):127-136.

Developing an Evidence-Based Practice

INTRODUCTION

This chapter pulls together many of the Evidence-Based Practice Tips that have been included in the previous 18 chapters. Again, as has been stressed throughout the text, you need to practice these activities and skills several times to be confident. Just keep working—your confidence will grow, and as your confidence grows, so will your competence.

LEARNING OUTCOMES

On completion of this chapter, the student should be able to do the following:

- Differentiate among conduct of nursing research, research utilization, and evidence-based practice.
- Describe the steps of evidence-based practice.
- Identify three barriers to evidence-based practice and strategies to address each barrier.
- List three sources for finding evidence.
- Describe strategies for implementing evidence-based practice changes.
- Identify steps for evaluating an evidence-based change in practice.
- Use research findings and other forms of evidence to improve the quality of care.

Activity 1

Following are short descriptions of RN activities related to research. Each can be categorized as one of the following:

A. Conduct of research
B. Dissemination of research findings
C. Research utilization
D. Evidence-based practice

Place the letter (A, B, C, D) that best describes each activity in the space provided.

1. _____ Mabel submits an article to the agency's in-house practice newsletter.

2. _____ Millicent and Margy are comparing two types of dressings for postop incisions.

3. _____ Mark has read about an intervention that will reduce the pain associated with the injection of a particular medication. After reviewing all of the variables, he decides that trying the intervention would be a good idea and proceeds to develop an implementation plan.

4. _____ Marie has been working with a faculty member on an independent study project. The two of them have decided to publish the results of their work.

5. _____ A group of students have been meeting twice a month in a journal club. They have developed a specific patient care question and plan to have care guidelines developed by the end of the year.

6. _____ Michael had developed a plan of care for Mr. Xavier using the findings from several studies and one meta-analysis. When he presented the plan to the client, Mr. Xavier declined. He stated that he needed more control than what the plan would allow. Michael went back to the drawing board.

7. _____ Marissa asked her classmates to taste chocolate chip cookies from three different recipes. She created a poster presentation to share the results of this taste test survey with the class.

Activity 2

Fill in the blanks with the appropriate word(s) from the text.

1. _____-driven evidence influences thinking, but not necessarily action.

2. The organizational perspective of evidence-based practice leads to the development of evidence-based _____ and _____.

3. The three approaches that can guide an organization as it moves toward evidence-based practice are:

   a.

   b.

   c.

4. A _____ trigger is one that arises when staff members interact directly with patients or with direct care-related situations.

5. A key individual (or group of individuals) who will be affected by the implementation of evidence-based practices and who are critical to successful implementation is known as a _____.

6. What does the acronym PICO stand for? _____

7. A group working on a review of evidence must agree on:

   a.

   b.

   c.

8. A summary table is very useful when one is getting ready to write a _____ of the research.

Activity 3

Number the following steps of evidence-based practice in the correct sequence. Use the number "1" for the first step.

a. _____   Selection of a topic

b. _____   Choose a scheme for grading the evidence

c. _____   Critique of research

d. _____   Implement the practice change

e. _____   Evaluate the use of the EBP

f. _____   Forming a team

g. _____   Critique EBP guidelines

h. _____   Delineate EBP recommendations

i. _____   Develop in detail the EBP

j. _____   Evidence retrieval

k. _____   Synthesis of research

l. _____   Decide to change practice

Activity 4

The creation of a procedure or a process that is evidence-based is not enough to establish the practice. The organization (or the unit of an organization) must create a culture that embraces EBP. The text described four building blocks that can help create this culture. List them below.

1.

2.

3.

4.

Now, think about yourself as an RN new to an agency. What actions can you take in each of the four areas you listed to facilitate EBP? There can be several for each building block.

5.

6.

7.

8.

☀ Activity 5: Evidence-Based Practice/Web-Based Activity

Go to the website http://www.joannabriggs.edu.au/about/home.php and click on "What's new at JBI?" Scroll down to March 2005 and click on the first article, "The JBI Best Practice Info Sheet (BPIS) 'Nurse Led Cardiac Clinics for Adults with Coronary Heart Disease'." Read the "Grades of Recommendation" that is on the first page of the article (on the right-hand side of the page). Scroll down to "Recommendations."

1.   How were the grades used?

2.   Was this article published in the U.S.?

3.   Does the origin of the article influence the use of the review?

POST-TEST

1.   Which of the following best describes "translation science"?
   a.   Increased use of evidence-based practice
   b.   Improvement of the culture of an organization so evidence-based practice can flourish
   c.   Description of the attitudes toward evidence-based practices
   d.   Investigation of variables that influence adoption of evidence-based practices

2. Evidence-based practice includes which of the following?
   a. Findings from randomized clinical trials
   b. Opinions of experts
   c. Information from case reports and other scientific studies
   d. Patient values
   e. All of the above
   f. None of the above

3. The Iowa Model of Evidence-Based Practice is an example of a/an:
   a. Type of research design
   b. Example of an EBP *practice* model
   c. Set of practice guidelines
   d. Organizational model that uses research evidence

4. Stakeholders are:
   a. People who own part of the health care agency
   b. Key individuals who can facilitate or hinder the move to EBP
   c. Administrators of any health care agency
   d. Members of the team that develops EBP guidelines

5. Before reading and critiquing research in a given area, it is useful to read:
   a. General articles on the same subject to gain an understanding of the topic
   b. Systematic review articles; e.g., meta-analyses
   c. All of the relevant medical intervention articles
   d. What is available at the Agency for Healthcare Research and Quality

6. Critiquing research studies can be made more interesting by:
   a. Forming a journal club
   b. Making the critique a class project for graduate students
   c. Asking interested students to assist in the process
   d. A and B only
   e. All of the above

7. Education of staff is critical for the implementation of EBP. Which of the following have been the most useful in this educational exercise?
   a. Disseminating information to everyone in the agency
   b. All staff members critique the research that guides the EBP
   c. Opinion leaders discuss the value of the EBP with staff
   d. Competency testing

8. Evaluation of EBP is important. Both process and outcome components of EBP should be evaluated. Use a "P" to mark the following items that are part of process evaluation. Use an "O" to mark those items that describe outcome evaluation.

   a. _____   Are staff using the EBP in care delivery?

   b. _____   What barriers are staff encountering?

   c. _____   Need for baseline data

   d. _____   Difficulty in carrying out the EBP activities

   e. _____   Patient and/or family satisfaction with the specific care activities

   f. _____   The cost of the EBP

Please check with your instructor for the answers to the post-test.

REFERENCE

The Joanna Briggs Institute. Accessed July 21, 2005 from http://www.joannabriggs.edu.au/about/home.php.

20 Tools for Applying Evidence to Practice

INTRODUCTION

The tools that you need to apply available evidence to your practice require you to think, ask questions, and get to know your local librarian very well. Practitioners face two major obstacles in applying available evidence to practice.

The first obstacle is finding the literature. The Internet has made this task easier and more difficult at the same time. It is easier because you don't have to get to the library before it closes; you can simply turn on your computer and log onto the Internet. Internet searches can yield millions of pieces of literature, which is why the Internet has made searching for appropriate articles more difficult: there is simply too much to search. The second obstacle is thinking through the analytical strategies that allow you to determine the usefulness of a given study or group of studies.

Both obstacles can be overcome. Help in searching the literature is available from your nearest health science librarian. Learning the analytical tools can be accomplished by thoroughly reading one study a month. Find a study in your clinical area of interest (the librarian can help). Pull out the textbook. Use the analytical strategies (tools) presented in Chapter 20 of the text and work until you understand how much faith you can place in this particular study.

LEARNING OUTCOMES

On completion of this chapter, the student should be able to do the following:

- Identify the key elements of a focused clinical question.
- Discuss the use of databases to search the literature.
- Learn how to screen an article for relevance and credibility.
- Evaluate study results and apply the findings to individual patients.
- Learn how to make clinical decisions based on evidence from the literature.

169

Activity 1

In each of the following scenarios, identify the relevant components of the mnemonic "PICO."

1. Janice is an RN on a pediatric unit that encourages parents to spend nights in the hospital room with their ill child. She has noticed that fewer parents are staying overnight since the in-room recliners have been replaced by Convert-A-Beds. Assume Janice decides to develop a focused clinical question.

   P _____

   I _____

   C _____

   O _____

2. Sam is an RN on a hemodialysis unit. Patients are provided verbal instruction about diet and fluid restrictions, but 81% of patients have trouble following the dietary restrictions and 75% of patients have difficulty in following the fluid restrictions.

   P _____

   I _____

   C _____

   O _____

3. Sharon is a school nurse. The concern about overweight children has led the school board to consider eliminating vending machines (snacks and soft drinks) from the schools in the district.

   P _____

   I _____

   C _____

   O _____

Activity 2

To help you overcome the first obstacle in applying evidence to practice—finding the studies that you need (and want) to read—you need to meet your health science librarian. Choose one of the activities below.

1. Go to the library on your campus and ask someone at the information desk where you can find the health science librarian. (University librarians have expertise in specific areas. One of the librarians will be responsible for health science areas.) When you locate the

health science librarian, introduce yourself and ask the librarian about the hours of availability. You also may want to ask whether the library provides sessions on "How to use your library to…" It is not uncommon for libraries to provide sessions specifically related to searching Lexis-Nexus or the Cochrane Library.

2. Go to the university's website and find the link to the library. Look for the staff information area and search for the health science librarian. E-mail this individual and ask the same questions you would ask if you were in the library (as outlined in option a).

Activity 3

There were five evidence-based tools discussed in Chapter 20. There are specific concepts and techniques associated with each tool. Place each word from the list in this activity with its appropriate evidence-based tool.

librarian	PICO	screening questions
therapy studies	diagnosis studies	information literacy
screening questions	meta analysis	confidence intervals
relative risk reduction	likelihood ratios	harm articles

Tool #1: Asking a focused clinical question _____

_____

Tool #2: Searching the literature _____

_____

Tool #3: Screening your findings _____

_____

Tool #4: Appraise each article's findings _____

_____

Tool #5: Applying the findings _____

_____

Activity 4

In this activity you will find several scenarios. Each will provide a description of a relevant clinical concern. They are not developed to the level of a PICO, but enough information is provided that you can begin to think about what clinical category would best fit. Your task is to specify which of the four clinical categories would fit each scenario.

First, list the four clinical categories.

1. _____

2. _____

3. _____

4. _____

Next, match the clinical category to the scenario.

5. Use of alcohol-based solution by RNs versus handwashing with antiseptic soap and bacterial count on hands.

6. Diet #1 was more effective than Diet #2 in reducing coronary artery disease risk factors.

7. Nurse visitation for adolescent mothers and rates of morbidity, unintentional injuries, and hospitalizations in their children in the first five years of life.

8. The role of individualized information in facilitating treatment decision-making regarding prostate cancer in men and their partners.

9. Milk and soft drink consumption in childhood and adolescence affects bone density later in life.

10. Confucian influences on HIV-positive partners and their decision to reproduce.

11. A new blood test is available to detect Alzheimer's disease.

12. Babies exposed to differing levels of cocaine before birth have learning difficulties.

Activity 5: Web-Based Activity

Go to the website http://www.cochrane.org. In the far right-hand column, click on "browse systematic reviews."

1. Scroll down and read about how you can gain access to the systematic reviews. What is required?

2. Go to the top of the page and click on "new/updated abstracts." What shows up? Click on one of the listed titles. What appears then?

3. Click on "NeLH little gems." Read the one entitled "Brief debriefing: Doesn't help, might harm." Would you change your practice based on this "little gem"? Read a few more that you find interesting.

4. Now go talk to the health science librarian and ask about gaining access to the systematic reviews of the Cochrane Library. What did you learn?

POST-TEST

Determine whether each of the following statements is True (T) or False (F). If an item is False, revise it to make it a True statement.

1. _____ An experimental or quasiexperimental study design is usually used for the diagnosis category of clinical concern.

2. _____ Articles should be screened to determine if the setting and sample in the study are similar to my clinical situation.

3. _____ Dichotomous variables are also known as outcomes.

4. _____ A confidence interval can provide the reader information about the statistical significance of the findings.

5. _____ *Specificity* is the term used to describe the proportion of individuals with a disease who test positive for it.

6. _____ The OR is a measure of association.

7. _____ Every study included in a meta-analysis is read by all members of the EBP team.

8. _____ Blobbogram is a new type of bubble gum.

9. _____ A meta-analysis synthesizes findings across many research studies.

Please check with your instructor for the answers to the posttest.

REFERENCE

The Cochrane Collaboration. Accessed July 21, 2005 from http://www.cochrane.org.

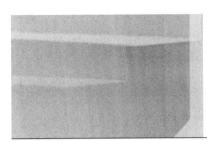

Answer Key

CHAPTER 1

Activity 1
1. c
2. b
3. d
4. a
5. g
6. e
7. f

Activity 2
1. D
2. B
3. C
4. D
5. A
6. B
7. A
8. C
9. B

Activity 3
1. a. EdD, RN, FAAN; PhD, RN; PhD, RN; PhD; PhD, RN, CS; PhD, RN; BMus
   b. PhD, RN, FAAN; DNS, RN; PhD, RN, FAAN; MN, RN; MD; DNS, RN, FAAN
   c. PhD, RN, CCRN; PhD, RN, FAAN; DNSc, RN
   d. PhD, RN; MD, FRCSC, FACS; MD, FRCSC, FACS; PhD, RN
2. a. Yes; Yes; Yes; Yes
   b. **Appendix A:** Authors Koniak-Griffin, Verzemnieks, Anderson, Brecht, Lesser, & Kim are all doctorally prepared and would obviously be more than qualified to design and implement the study. Turner-Pluta is not doctorally prepared and her role is as an administrative analyst.

Appendix B: Van Cleve, Bossert, Beecroft, Alvarez & Savedra are all doctorally prepared and would be more than qualified to design and implement the study. Adlard is master's prepared and would be appropriate to assist with the design and implementation of the study.

Appendix C: Plach, Stevens, & Moss are all doctorally prepared and would be more than qualified to design and implement the study.

Appendix D: Davison, Goldenberg, Gleave, & Degner are all doctorally prepared and would be more than qualified to design and implement the study.

c. **Appendix A:** The Koniak-Griffin et al. study was funded by grants from NINR and the Office of Research on Women's Health.

Appendix B: The Van Cleve et al. study was funded by a grant from NINR.

Appendix C: The Plach, Stevens, & Moss study was funded in part by a grant from the University of Wisconsin-Oshkosh Faculty Development Program.

Appendix D: The Davison et al. study was funded by the Prostate Cancer Research Initiative, the National Cancer Institute of Canada, and a Scholar Award from Vancouver General Hospital.

Activity 4

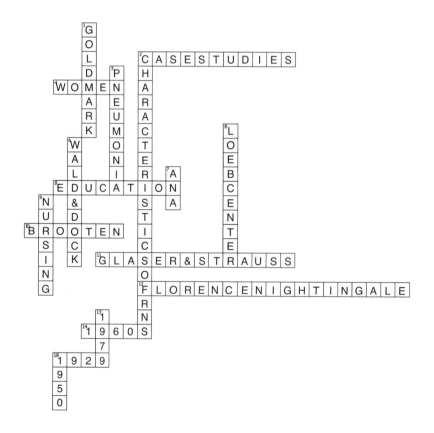

Activity 5
a. Continuing to conduct research on the topic of abuse in women
b. Developing theoretical perspectives
c. Conducting synthesis conferences discussing the area of abuse of women
d. Using nursing research studies to assist in legislative change

Activity 6
1. In order to base your practice on scientific evidence gained through research, you must first understand the research process. Then you need to know how to critique research in order to decide whether particular studies and their results have enough merit to change your practice.
2. Depth in nursing science will occur when a sufficient number of nurse researchers replicate and have consistent findings in a substantive area of inquiry. It is important that each study builds on prior studies, adding new variables or questions as the need arises.
3. If, for instance, your area of practice is psychiatric/mental health nursing with an emphasis on chemical dependency, you would like research findings demonstrating that nursing interventions related to "knowledge deficit regarding addiction" have an effect on the outcome of increased sobriety time for the addict or alcoholic.

CHAPTER 2

Activity 1
1. rational
2. active; inner
3. the point of view of the writer
4. nursing
5. three (or four)

Activity 2
1. b
2. b
3. a
4. b
5. a
6. a

Activity 3
1. a. Preliminary understanding
   b. Comprehensive understanding
   c. Analysis understanding
   d. Synthesis understanding
2. a. Read the article for the fourth time.
   b. Review your notes on the copy.

    c.   Summarize study in your own words.

    d.   Complete one handwritten 5 x 8 card per study.

    e.   Staple the summary to the top of copied article.

Activity 4

1. Yes
2. No
3. No
4. Yes
5. Yes [Instruments used include the: 1) Patient Information Program, 2) Spielberger State Anxiety Inventory, and 3) Center for Epidemiologic Studies Depression Scale]
6. Yes
7. Yes

    Summary: I would categorize this study as quantitative. It meets 5 of the 7 criteria listed. It is a quasiexperimental, one-group, pretest/post-test design.

Activity 5

Go to the reference section and locate the article by Plach, Napholz, & Kelber found in *Health Care for Women International.*

Activity 6

Answers for this activity will vary.

Activity 7

1. The Van Cleve et al. study (2004) falls into Level VI because of its descriptive design, while the Davison et al. study (2003) falls into Level III because of its quasiexperimental design. Note, however, that it is only one study without a control group, so it doesn't fit easily into the model and could also be labeled at Level VI.
2. Answers for this activity will vary depending on the reasearch article chosen.

CHAPTER 3

Activity 1

1. e
2. b
3. d
4. a
5. c

Activity 2

1. Yes; Yes; Yes; Yes
2. No; No; Yes; Yes
3. Yes; No; Yes; Yes

Activity 3
1. a. CRTs
   b. Birth defects
2. a. Birth defects
   b. Independence/dependence conflicts
3. a. White wine
   b. Serum cholesterol level
4. a. Type of recording
   b. Patient care
5. a. Profession (MD or RN)
   b. Extended-role concept of RNs
6. a. Sex, age, height, weight
   b. Physiologic outcomes

Activity 4
1. H_R, DH
2. H_R, DH
3. RQ
4. H_R, DH
5. H_R, NDH
6. RP

Activity 5
1. RQ: Does the use of CRTs by pregnant women influence the incidence of birth defects?
   Ho: The use of CRTs by pregnant women has no effect on the incidence of birth defects.
2. DH: As is in the chapter.
   NDH: There is a difference in the number of independence/dependence conflicts between individuals with and without birth defects.
   H_R: As is.
   RQ: Do individuals with birth defects have a higher incidence of independence/dependence conflicts than those without birth defects?
   Ho: There is no difference in incidence of independence/dependence conflicts between individuals with and without birth defects.
3. DH: There is a positive relationship between daily moderate consumption of white wine and serum cholesterol levels.
   NDH: Daily moderate consumption of white wine influences serum cholesterol levels.
   H_R: There is a relationship between daily moderate consumption of white wine and serum cholesterol levels.
   RQ: As is.
   Ho: There is no relationship between daily moderate consumption of white wine and serum cholesterol levels.

Activity 6
1. a. Yes
   b. Yes; IV-SPID; DV-dressing independence
   c. Yes
   d. Yes
   e. Yes
   f. Yes
   g. Yes
2. a. Yes
   b. Yes
   c. Yes
   d. Yes
   e. Yes
   f. Yes
   g. Yes

Activity 7
1. a. There is probably not enough time for the student to design and conduct this study. It will take a considerable amount of time to conceptualize this problem and would be a more appropriate study for a doctoral thesis where a student usually has 3 years to resolve a problem. During the first year of doctoral study, the student could work on refining the problem in design classes, and then have a full 1 to 2 years to conduct the study, analyze the data, and complete the write-up.
   b. This is difficult to answer based on the information given in the brief scenario. Because the nurse has identified it as a problem, one would assume he or she is aware of a unit where this change is occurring; whether the nurse would be able to gain access to that unit to conduct research is an unknown until he or she sends a letter and asks permission of the setting and the setting's Institutional Review Board.
   c. The lack of experience of the researcher is probably the greatest impediment to conducting this study. It will take a very experienced and knowledgeable researcher to determine which variables to study and to develop a study design that will give meaningful answers to this question. This is probably why the definitive study in this area has not yet been done.
   d. No ethical issues inherent in conducting this study are foreseen.
2. Yes. The significance would be related to the relationship between cost of patient care technicians (PCTs) and registered nurses (PCTs are less costly), and patient outcomes in terms of satisfaction, morbidity, and mortality. Remember that one would need to assume that a thorough literature review did not provide an answer.

Activity 8
The problem statement poses the question the researcher is asking. The hypothesis attempts to answer the question posed by the research problem. The problem statement does not predict a relationship between two or more variables.

CHAPTER 4

Activity 1
1. research
2. education
3. research; practice
4. theory

Activity 2
1. f
2. c
3. a
4. e
5. d
6. c
7. b

Activity 3
1. D
2. C
3. D
4. D
5. C
6. D

Activity 4
Any of the following scholarly nursing journals may be listed:
Advances in Nursing
AORN Journal
Applied Nursing Research
Archives of Psychiatric Nursing
Computers in Nursing
Heart & Lung
Holistic Nursing Practice
Image: Journal of Nursing Scholarship
Journal of Professional Nursing
Journal of Nursing Education
NACOG
Nurse Educator
Nursing Diagnosis
Nursing & Health Care
Nursing Research
Nursing Science Quarterly
Research in Nursing & Health

Scholarly Inquiry for Nursing Practice
Western Journal of Nursing Research

Activity 5
1. a. Review of literature
   b. Background literature review
2. a. No
   b. Yes, these authors uncover a gap in prior research. They note that although there has been much research on the patient's pain with cancer, it has focused almost exclusively on the procedure-related pain. Very little research has been conducted to increase knowledge about pain over time as related by children.
3. Yes, the majority of the references are current ranging from the mid-1990s to 2002. It does read like a well-designed research proposal. The first cited research study on the topic was in 1983. It reported that health promotion interventions for adolescent mothers and their children continued to have positive outcomes not evident until a year or more after the intervention program ended. A 15-year longitudinal study examined maternal and child outcomes in a nurse home visitation intervention program (studies cited from 1986-1997). The studies cited in the 1990s reported variables and positive outcomes with home intervention programs to improve maternal child health. The current research study is a continuation of the author's previous work (2000, 2003) of an early intervention program (EIP) with adolescent mothers. The new variable in this research examined the effects of an intensive EIP versus the traditional PHN care.

Activity 6
1. a. S
   b. P
   c. S
   d. S
   e. P
   f. P
   g. P
2. False
3. False
4. True
5. b; MEDLINE does not contain all nursing references like CINAHL
6. True
7. True
8. False

Activity 7
1. C; P
2. D; P
3. D; P

4. D; S
5. D; P

Activity 8

1. What is the source of the material?
   (*Note:* Look at the last term in the URL address to find the organizational name [it is three letters long]; possibilities include: *.com* for commercial organization, *.edu* for educational institution, *.gov* for government body, *.int* for international organization, *.mil* for U.S. military, *.net* for networking organization, and *.org* for anything else. Information gathered from an *.edu* or *.gov* source are most reliable, such as www.ncbi.nlm.nih.gov which takes you to the Pub Med Query source for MEDLINE at the U.S. National Library of Medicine.
2. Is the source a well-respected medical or nursing institution or a federal agency, or is the source an individual putting out his or her own opinion? Critique the source.
3. Is the name of the researcher(s) and their degrees given?
4. Is there a mechanism given to obtain further information about the study or the information presented?
5. Is enough data given in the web publication to make a critical analysis about the material? (*Note:* Remember, in a refereed, professional journal, usually three independent nursing experts in the field have reviewed the article in a blind review process to determine that this material merits publication.)

CHAPTER 5

Activity 1

1. Inductive thinking moves from the particular to the general (or conclusions are developed from specific observations)
   Deductive thinking moves from the general to the particular (or predictions are developed from known relationships)
2. a. Inductive
   b. Deductive
3. Observations will vary. If you were able to write a general statement about "headache pain," you used inductive thinking and probably wrote something like:

   X (grimacing) X (rubbing temples) X (grumpy) = indications of headache pain.

   If you were unable to write a general statement, it could be that you do not know anyone who has headaches, so you don't have a database.

Activity 2

1. a. Learned helplessness, self-esteem, depression, health practices, homeless (*Note:* You would also be correct if you listed women.)
   b. Illness uncertainty, stress, coping, emotional well-being, clinical drug trial
   c. Social support, intervention, pregnancy, pregnancy outcome, lower income, African-American
   d. Violent behavior, nonviolent behavior, behavior, vulnerable, inner-city youths

e. Verbal abuse, staff nurses, physicians, stress coping (*Note:* Prevalence and consequences may also be listed as consequences, especially if you think of them as capturing an idea.)

2. a. "Beauty" is a concept. "Nursing diagnosis" is a construct.
   b. "Beauty" and "nursing diagnosis" are similar in that both describe an abstraction. Both terms describe some notion that people want to be able to discuss, think about, or use without spending hours describing what is meant.
   c. The terms are different in one important dimension. "Beauty" is a concept that all people recognize, although the precise characteristics of beauty may vary from person to person. The construct "nursing diagnosis" is an abstraction that has been created by a specific discipline to explain a concept unique to that discipline. All disciplines, especially researchers within a given discipline, create constructs to structure their world of study.

3. Answers will vary. An argument could be made for the following as constructs: illness uncertainty, social support intervention, and verbal abuse.

4. Answers will vary.

Activity 3

1. The two major concepts are discharge planning and patient/caregiver outcome measures. Each of these was operationally defined as follows:
   Discharge planning: One of two types—usual discharge planning procedures or a professional-patient partnership model of discharge planning.
   Patient outcomes: Defined as perceived health, client satisfaction, caregiver's response to caregiving, and resource use. These definitions are strengthened by the information in Table 2.

2. The concepts of this study were hope and fear. Given the qualitative nature of this study, precise definitions would not be expected. The intent of this study is to more clearly articulate the concept.

3. The major concepts in this study are trait anger, state anger, general well-being, symptom patterns, vigor, and inclination to change.
   Trait anger: Defined as responses to items on the Spielberger Trait Anger Scale that assess how angry one generally feels.
   State anger: Defined as responses to items on the Spielberger State Anger Scale that assess how angry one is feeling right now.
   General well-being: Defined as responses to items on the Adolescent General Well-Being Questionnaire that assesses the social, physical, and mental dimensions of well-being.
   Symptom patterns: Defined as responses to items on the Symptom Pattern Scale that measure physical, psychological, and psychosomatic manifestations of psychological distress.
   Vigor: Defined as responses to items on the Vigor subscale of the Profile of Mood States that assesses vigor.
   Inclination to change: Defined as responses to items on the change subscale of the Personality Research Form E that assesses inclination to change.

4. The major concepts in this study are pile-up, existing and new resources, perception of stressors, and adaptation.

    Pile-up: Defined as family strains and as responses to items on the Family Inventory of Life Events and Changes that assesses family stress variables with the ability to assess the pile-up events.

    Existing and new resources: Defined as social support and coping. Social support is defined as responses to items on the Norbeck Social Support questionnaire that evaluates a person's social support network. Coping is defined as responses to items on the Coping Health Inventory for Parents that assesses parent's coping responses in the management of family life when a child is seriously ill.

    Perception of stressor: Defined as responses to items on the Parent Perception of Uncertainty Scale that assesses a parent's perception of uncertainty as a stress. Also defined as responses to the Profile of Mood States that assesses a person's level of mood and subjective affect.

    Family adaptation: Defined as responses to items on the McMaster's Family Assessment Device that assesses family functioning and is used to measure family adaptation.

Activity 4

1. a. 4
    b. 5
    c. 6
    d. 4
    e. 5 or 3
    f. 3
    g. 6
    h. 1
    i. 2
2. a. Anger
    b. i. Anger is a major concern of early adolescents and it has not been studied much in this population.
        ii. There is a lack of studies on positive outcomes of anger in early adolescents.
        iii. Trait anger and state anger are defined by Spielberger and colleagues.
        iv. Personality traits have an impact on the way people are predisposed to behave or act in a certain way.
        v. Described variables in the model and how they relate to one another.
        vi. Anger can be exhibited as symptom patterns in adolescents.
    c. Deductive
    d. Yes
    e. A conceptual model

Activity 5

Critiquing Grid

		Well Done	OK	Needs Help	Not Applicable
1.	Theoretical rationale was clearly identified (Could I find it?)	K; V; D		P	
2.	The information in the theoretical component matches what the researchers are studying	K;V; D		P	
3.	Concepts:				
	a. Conceptual definition(s) found	K;V; D		P	
	b. Conceptual definition(s) clear	K; V; D;		P	
	c. Operational definition(s) found	K; V; D		P	
	d. Operational definition(s) clear	K; V; D		P	
4.	Enough literature was reviewed:				
	a. For an expert in the area	K; V; D		P	
	b. For a nurse with some knowledge	K; V; D		P	
	c. For a nurse reading outside of area of specialty or interest	K; V; D	P		
5.	Thinking of researcher:				
	a. Can be followed through theoretical material to hypotheses or questions	K; V; D		P	
	b. Makes sense	K; V; D		P	
6.	Relationships among propositions clearly stated	D	K; V	P	
7.	Theory:				
	a. Borrowed	V; D			K;P
	b. Concepts/data related to nursing	K;V;P;D			
8.	Findings related back to theoretical base (I can find each concept from the theory section discussed in the "Results" section of the report.)	V; D	K	P	

Note: As you see, it is not easy to make unequivocal statements about every criterion. Some criteria do not fit one study as well as they fit another study. The use of a grid like the one above is a start in your critical thinking. It makes sure that you have addressed the same areas for each study. You then have to put this information together with your evaluation of the other pieces of the study to make the final critical judgment of the quality of the specific study.

CHAPTER 6

Activity 1

1. a. Quantitative research: The quantitative approach to research is based in the belief that we can best understand humans and their behavior by taking the human apart. We study specific characteristics one at a time. We measure each one as we go in the hopes that we can understand each characteristic in a clear and context-free manner. Once we clearly understand all of the pieces, we can put them together and understand the whole. Quantitative studies rely much more heavily on preselected instruments, collect lots of data, and answer questions through the analysis of numbers that represent those characteristics.

    b. Qualitative research: The qualitative approach to research is an accepted way to discover knowledge that uses naturalistic approaches to learn about human phenomena. This method of research is grounded in the social sciences and provides nurses with ways to better understand the lived experience and human processes that surround health and illness.

2. a. Karl Popper's (1902-1994) leading philosophical perspective had to do with methodological views called *falsification*. Falsification is the idea that science advances by unjustified or unfounded presumptions that are then liberally criticized by the scientific world. Theories that are falsifiable can expand knowledge by improving our control about errors in judgment as to what is true or false about the world. Theories that are falsifiable are only problems to clear thinking and act like logjams in the stream of knowledge. Popper thought that while a theory could be unscientific (unfalsifiable), it could still be enlightening and able to become falsified or scientific with further refinement. Popper thought that a major problem in the philosophy of science was determining differences between what is scientific and what comprises nonscience. From this perspective, a genuine test of scientific theory is an attempt to refute or falsify it. Although a theory has stood for a long time and appears to be good science, it is still possible that error exists and at some later time the theory may be falsified.

    Edmund Husserl (1859-1939) initially pursued interests in attempts to describe a psychological foundation of arithmetic. However, when his work was formally criticized, he turned away from psychology and turned to philosophy. Husserl is known for developing the philosophical method called *phenomenology*. His first phenomenological work, entitled *Logical Investigations*, was published in two volumes. His philosophy is based upon the study of consciousness that a speaker presents or "gives voice to" in response to a proposition in question. Husserl describes these units of consciousness as *intentional acts* or *intentional experiences*. Husserl argued that a more precise study of discrete phenomena, ideas, and simple events was possible. Phenomenology could be described as an awareness of matter can be clearly disclosed in distinct ways and made known, visible, and be understood.

    Hans-Georg Gadamer (1900-2002) lived a very full life in his 102 years and is viewed as the key figure in the study of hermeneutics. Hermeneutic thinking seeks to investigate the basic structures of factual existence that allows self-disclosure to occur. He argued that in order for things to be understood about some situation, object, behavior, one must have prior understanding; otherwise it is impossible to have understanding. In order for us to have understanding, we must already find ourselves 'in' the world 'along with' that which is to be understood. Gadamer encouraged individuals "to go back to the things themselves" and recover the original awareness. Thus, hermeneutics can be understood as the attempt to "make explicit" the structure of such situatedness. In Gadamer's way of thinking, it is a matter of "laying bare" a structure with which we are already familiar and, in this way, hermeneutics becomes one with phenomenology.

b. Martin Heidegger (1889-1976), a German philosopher, developed the ideas of existential phenomenology. This philosophical perspective explores the essential question: What is it to be? Humans are continually affected by the world they live in and struggle with time, objects, daily routines, and the behaviors of others. Heidegger's most influential work is entitled *Being and Time* (1927, translated to English in 1962). He believed that the existence of the physical body came before the fundamental nature of self, but at some point a being becomes aware of its own existence and a new essence is formed. Human being is comprised of concern, being-toward death, existence, and moods. Heidegger's philosophy is an effort to comprehend the meaning of "being" in its general and concrete forms, and a conception of human existence as active participation "being there" in the world.

Activity 2

a. Epistemology: A branch of philosophy that deals with what we know as truth or knowledge and includes its origins, limits, and nature.

b. Ontology: A branch of philosophy that studies the nature of being or existence.

c. Context: The place where something occurs and can include physical place, cultural beliefs, and life experience.

d. Paradigm: From the Greek word meaning "pattern," it has come to describe how a person or a group of people think about the world.

e. Constructivism: The basis for naturalistic (qualitative) research which is guided by the ontological perspective and suggests that many realities exist rather than only a single reality.

f. Postpositivism: Truth is sought through replicable observations based upon the premise that a single reality exists.

Activity 3

Here is an example of how a researcher might view the problem of pain management differently based upon whether he or she assumed a constructivist or postpositivistic perspective.

If pain management associated with cancer is considered using a postpositivistic paradigm, the approach used might be to measure the physiologic nature of pain mechanisms or the efficacy of a specific drug protocol versus an alternative therapy. In this case, it is highly likely that the researcher would select a research design with several groups that include a control group. The purpose would be to investigate the effects of various treatments on pain relief. The researcher may identify a large number of study participants that includes participant eligibility based upon gender, race, ethnicity, and age in order to identify whether these variables make a difference in pain relief. However, if one chooses to use a constructivist approach to investigate the problem, then the number of participants would likely be far smaller and may even be more homogenous in nature. For example, the investigator may want to describe the experience of pain management in black women. The purpose of the study might be to explain the realities of living with cancer pain in women using alternative therapies.

Activity 4

1. a. Grounded theory: A research method that enables the investigator to discover a theory from systematically obtained data. The data comes from the observations of the participants being studied. The purpose of this research is to generate theory.
    b. Case study: A research method that provides an in-depth description of the phenomena of interest to the investigator. Data for case studies may come from a variety of sources. This research method provides a way to study complex phenomena that are poorly understood.
    c. Phenomenological research: A research method that examines naturalistic experiences as they are lived and understood as reality by human beings. Researchers examine phenomena that are of special interest to nursing. The goal of this research method is to understand experience from the perspective of those having the experience.
    d. Ethnographic research: A research method initially developed by anthropologists to study the ways human beings react within or experience a cultural setting. The goal of this research method is to combine the emic (insider) with the etic (outsider) perspective. Nurses have used an adaptation called *ethnomethod* to study health and illness within a variety of cultural contexts.
2. (Your answers may not be identical, but may include similar ideas.)
    a. Grounded theory: This research method is useful for nurses as they search for knowledge about social behaviors. Methods often used in this type of research are unstructured interviews or conversation with a purpose. Data are analyzed using abstract categories until saturation is reached or no new information is being discovered.
    b. Case study: This research method uses in-depth interviews with participants and key informants, medical record reviews, observation, and excerpts from personal diaries or writings. Case studies in a way are life histories that enable the investigator to gain knowledge as he or she studies a person or phenomena of concern over a long period of time. Case study designs must have five components: (a) the research question(s), (b) its propositions, (c) its unit(s) of analysis, (d) a determination of how data are linked to the propositions, and (e) criteria to interpret the findings.
    c. Phenomenological research: Phenomenology entails listening and truly hearing what people are saying in order to understand the lived experience from the perspective of the other. This type of research requires an attitude of inquiry that includes radical openness and extreme attentiveness to the world we live in. In order for one to do this type of research, the investigator must bracket or put aside his or her experience.
    d. Ethnographic research: The goal of ethnographic research is to look for patterns, themes, connections, and relationships that have meanings for the people involved. Questions of interest in the ethnographic process are: What is this? What is happening in this subculture? In order to gain access and complete an ethnographic study, the

researcher usually identifies key informants or "insiders" who can provide access to others who can help tell the story.

Activity 5: Web-Based Activity

(In order to complete this activity, you must read the essay entitled "How can we argue for evidence in nursing?" at http://www.contemporarynurse.com/11.1/11-1p5.htm.)

Consider what kinds of evidence you might need to adequately care for all the needs of a young woman with type 1 diabetes who has suffered the complications of blindness and kidney failure, and spends three days a week associating with very ill elderly individuals on dialysis. Although much of her care may be related to the hemodialysis and physiologic responses of her body to this medical procedure, nurses are also concerned about the holistic needs of patients. What kinds of evidence do you think might be needed to enable a nurse to provide optimal or excellent care for this client? What kinds of evidence might you need to know about caregivers, the family household, adjusting to blindness, socialization needs, and other aspects of abilities to accomplish activities of daily living? What kinds of contributions might researchers using qualitative methods make to identify the kinds of interventions needed? The evidence that nurses need to provide optimal nursing care for the whole person may not be fully provided through quantitative studies. Qualitative research that explores the behavioral, emotional, and spiritual aspects of living with illness is needed so that we can truly identify what might be the best nursing approaches for meeting specific care needs. This is an area where nurses will make large contributions in the next few decades.

CHAPTER 7

Activity 1

1. a. scientific; artistic
    b. natural settings
    c. day-to-day life
    d. lived experience
    e. less
    f. everyday living; human uniqueness
    g. research question
    h. fit
2. a. D
    b. A
    c. C
    d. F
    e. B
    f. I
    g. J
    h. G
    i. E
    j. H

3. a. Element 1: Identifying the phenomenon
    1. Phenomenology: Study of day-to-day existence for a particular group of people
    2. Grounded theory method: Interested in social processes from perspective of human interactions.
    3. Ethnography: Study of the complex cultural aspects related to a phenomenon.
    4. Historical research: An approach for understanding a past event.
    5. Case study: A focus on an individual, family, community, an organization, or some other complex phenomenon.
    6. Community-based participatory research: A systematic study or assessment of a community to plan context-appropriate action.
  b. Element 2: Structuring the study
    1. Phenomenology: Query the lived experience, research perspective is bracketed, sample has either lived or is living the experience being investigated.
    2. Grounded theory: Questions address basic social processes and tend to be action-oriented; researcher brings some knowledge of the literature but exhaustive review is not done prior to beginning the research. The researcher has concerns about contextual values and the data are the essence of the theory that emerges. The sample would be participants who have had experience with the circumstances, events, or incidents being studied.
    3. Ethnography: Questions are about lifeways or patterns of behavior within a social or cultural context. Researcher attempts to make sense of world from insider's point of view. The researcher becomes the interpreter of events and tries to make sense and understand things from an emic point of view. Researchers do this by making their own beliefs explicit and set aside their own biases or assumptions in order to better understand a different world view. The sample often consists of key informants who have knowledge, status, and the communication skills needed to describe the phenomenon being studied.
    4. Historical: Questions are implicit and embedded in the phenomenon studied; researcher understands information without imposing interpretation. It is important for the researcher to clearly and carefully identify the event(s) being studied. Data used for the study may be of a primary or secondary nature.
    5. Case study: Questions about issues that serve as a foundation to uncover complexity and pursue understanding. The perspective of the researcher is reflected in the questions. Researchers may choose the most common cases or instead select the most unusual ones.
    6. Community-based participatory research: Questions in this form of research are framed around the ideas of "look." Look has to do with identification of the stakeholders and understanding the problems from their perspective.
  c. Element 3: Gathering the data
    1. Phenomenology: Written or oral data may be collected.
    2. Grounded theory: Collect data through audiotaped and transcribed interviews and skilled observations.
    3. Ethnography: Participant observation, immersion, informant interviews.
    4. Historical: Use of primary and secondary data sources.

     5. Case study: Use of interview, observations, document reviews, and other methods.

     6. Community-based participatory research: Seeks to engage stakeholders in discovering the answers to the community problems.

  d. Element 4: Analyzing the data

     1. Phenomenology: Move from the participant's description to the researcher's synthesis.

     2. Grounded theory: Data collection and analysis occur simultaneously, use theoretical sampling, constant comparative method, and axial coding.

     3. Ethnography: Data are collected and analyzed simultaneously, searching for symbolic categories.

     4. Historical: Analyze for importance and then validity (authenticity) and reliability.

     5. Case study: Reflecting and revising meanings.

     6. Community-based participatory research: This stage of research is the "think" phase and is where what has been learned is interpreted or analyzed. The research has the role of linking the ideas provided by the stakeholders in an understandable way so that evidence for specific ways to address the problem can be provided to the community group.

  e. Element 5: Describing the findings

     1. Phenomenology: A narrative elaboration of the lived experience.

     2. Grounded theory: Descriptive language to show theory connections to the data.

     3. Ethnography: Large quantities of data; provide examples from the data and propositions about relationships of phenomena.

     4. Historical: Well-synthesized chronicle.

     5. Case study: Chronologically developed cases, a story that describes case dimensions or vignettes that emphasize various aspects of the case.

     6. Community-based participatory research: Information obtained in earlier research stages sets the stage for community planning, implementation, and evaluation.

4. Your answers may vary based upon your personal interests. For example, a personal interest in the health behaviors of individuals and families in a culturally unique group might lead to the selection of an ethnographic method of investigation. This research method allows the investigator to explore multiple aspects of individual and family life, means of communication and behaviors, locations and substance of family households, the impact of the situated context where they reside, and other related factors. Understanding the health practices of a specific cultural group can be understood from emic and etic perspectives, ideas that may be similar or different. Data are collected through observation, interviews, identifying objects and their uses, and determining valuing associated with symbols, behaviors, and objects.

Activity 2

1. The main theme of the literature review was that people with rheumatoid arthritis suffer from symptoms that affect emotional and physical health and cause them to alter their lifestyle.

2. The literature review describes specific symptoms associated with rheumatoid arthritis that alter functional capacities and suggests ways these problems interfere over time with successful management of everyday life activities. The disease affects emotional feelings, ability to fulfill social roles, physical decline, and ideas about progressive disability. The authors make a case for understanding that rheumatoid arthritis increases women's vulnerability.

3. The larger study found that women who had rheumatoid arthritis and positive social role experiences had less depression and more purpose in life, despite physical difficulties, than those who did not have positive social role experiences. What this study did not explain was what comprised this social role experience. Thus, a follow-up qualitative study with a subset of the women in the earlier study was selected to more closely examine how fulfilling particular roles were found to be viewed. The study also allowed the investigators to explore the circumstances that made social role experiences positive ones. The quantitative study was not able to answer these questions.

Activity 3

1. The research design used in this study was not stated. It is generally believed by nurse researchers that the design of the study should be stated. The study uses a purposive sample, which might indicate phenomenology. However, the use of semi-structured interviews is not the data-collection method generally used with this design.

2. A purposive sample of 20 women was chosen from the original 156 women who had given permission to be contacted again. The sample was selected based upon length of time since diagnosis and age. The investigators wanted to select a sample that had lived with the illness for long enough to be able to describe what it was like. The researchers also wanted to include women in midlife and late life to learn more about levels of depression associated with the disease.

3. The procedures used to collect data in this study were semi-structured interviews mostly comprised of open-ended questions that lasted from 45 to 90 minutes. Interviews were mostly conducted in participant's homes. Interviews were taped and later transcribed verbatim.

4. Content analysis was used to find common patterns and themes. The data was coded twice. First level coding was to identify social roles, and second level coding was associated with the context and circumstances of positive role. Finally, categories were identified that represented the relationships among the themes. Trustworthiness and rigor were established by the use of three researchers collaborating and coming to consensus during the coding and analysis.

Activity 4

You may have some different ideas about the implications of this study for nursing practice, but here are a few things to consider:

Rheumatoid arthritis is a debilitating disease that leaves individuals feeling useless, sad, and angry. The unburdening of social responsibilities as the women grew older was a positive experience for them and also seemed to bring wisdom that made them more accepting of their conditions. Having more time free from social obligations meant that women were better able to tend to their own needs.

Living with rheumatoid arthritis was a process for these women that changed over time with adaptation occurring as they learned to balance the resources and demands associated with the illness. Nurses working with women who are experiencing rheumatoid arthritis may want to consider education of not only the woman with the disease, but also the spouse, partner, or other family members about ways they can provide support at different adult developmental stages. The availability of a support group or network may also be useful in providing the opportunity for the sharing of experiences. This disease, like many other chronic illnesses, is a concern that may be best addressed using family-centered care.

Activity 5

a. D
b. C
c. B
d. A
e. A
f. B
g. E
h. C
i. D
j. D
k. A
l. C
m. E
n. C
o. D
p. C
q. B
r. A
s. E
t. A (could also be true of B or C)
u. A (could also be true of B, C, or D)
v. C
w. D (could also be true of A or C)
x. C (could also be true of A)
y. B
z. C

Activity 6

The author has provided examples from her own experience, but you may want to consider this activity in relation to a research study you might like to conduct.

a. In a research study about family health (Denham 1999), the method selected to study the phenomenon was ethnography. The researcher wanted to identify clearer definitions about the family health concept and gain knowledge about the ways health was addressed within the family household. It was necessary to operate within the culture of the families included in the study. The use of key informants allowed the opportunity to learn about the community context as well as the health of selected families residing within the rural community.

An alternative method of study, phenomenology, was also considered as a possible method. Phenomenology could have been used to study the lived experience of family health. Case study could have been used to study family health in a single family over time. Historical methods might have been used to investigate the ways family health was interpreted over the last 100 years.

b. 1. The ways families define health.
    2. The ways individual health is influenced by family.
    3. The way individuals practice health behaviors on a daily basis within a family household.
c. How do families define and practice family health in their household setting?
d. Families each took part in four audiotaped interviews. Fifteen community informants served as key informants about family health in the community. Participant observation, journal, and field notes were also used as data-collection methods.
e. Study subjects were located with the assistance of key community informants and the use of snowball techniques. The subjects were eight rural Appalachian families with preschool children. A total of 39 family members and 15 community informants participated in the study.
f. Data analysis initially involved transcription of the interviews and the use of qualitative software and the use of content analysis to sort and identify themes in the large data set. The analysis included family cases, but constant comparative methods were used to contrast parents, children, and community informant data within and between families.
g. Subjects affirmed the importance of family in producing health, the role of mothers in providing care, the value of early childhood as a time when health behaviors are learned, and the value of the household production of health. Study findings identified that family health was largely a product of family context, family functioning, and family health routines. New knowledge pointed to the complex interactions among family and community that create dynamic and evolving patterns of family health. Family health routines were identified as a way to describe and discuss individual and family health behaviors.

As a nurse, the information in the study encourages one to think about where the focus of health teaching should occur. Using the medical model, the tendency is to focus on individuals and treat family members as the background of individual care. Patient-centered care is the focus of many health care providers. However, this study along with many others, suggests that family-centered care is needed. Increasing demands for caregivers suggest that the needs for inclusion of family are becoming greater and will only increase in the next decade. Given that individuals spend most of their time in the family household and only occasional amounts of time interacting with health care providers, an implication for nursing education is to find better ways to teach nurses about how to intervene and support individuals as they care for individual family members.

Activity 7: Web-Based Activity

Qualitative research provides many unique ways to add to nursing's body of knowledge as it supplies evidence related to the complex behavioral relationships between humans and humans with their environment. This activity is intended to expose you to the broad kinds of investigation being done using qualitative research.

a. Collaborative inquiry is a form of community-based participatory research or action research. Collaborative inquiry treats research as a form of learning and is defined by these authors as repeated episodes of reflection and action in which a group of peers strives to answer a question of importance to them.

b. Knowledge is constructed through repeated episodes of reflection and action. The investigators become co-inquirers and co-subjects in the process. Forming the collaborative group and assuring that investigators are passionate about investigating the phenomena of interest, are willing to collaborate in the process, and have skills needed for communication throughout the process are essential elements of this research form.

c. Pain is a common experience for human beings; however, human perceptions about pain vary from person to person and culture to culture. Findings from this study support findings from many other quantitative and qualitative studies. Thus, the body of evidence about the uniqueness of cultural experience is a constant reminder that nurses must not assume they understand the pain experience of others. The findings from this collaborative inquiry suggest that similarities and broad differences exist around the way pain is experienced and perceived across cultures. Clarifying these differences adds evidence for our thinking in both how we practice in clinical settings and how we teach new nurses about pain management.

CHAPTER 8

Activity 1

The primary theme of this first discussion of the findings describes the conflict that women experience as they feel the tug between their desire to fulfill social roles and the distress experienced when they fail to meet their expectations. These women with RA experienced a number of problems that affected most areas of their life and caused them to experience feelings of loss, inadequacy, and isolation.

Activity 2

1. This study emphasizes that the deleterious effects of RA on social roles and psychological activities are similar to what has been identified through other research. The adaptation process experienced by these women over time allows them to become more productive in managing their lives despite the constraints of the disease.

2. Over the course of the lifespan, women with RA have different role expectations; the unburdening of social obligation and role responsibilities with aging tends to be viewed positively. At different developmental stages, emotional and physical well-being may be viewed and experienced differently. Things that are important at one life point may be valued less at another. Findings suggest that nurses should take into consideration the

developmental life point of a woman before assuming some things about responses to social role expectations.

3. Ideas associated with feminist perspectives suggest that women in caregiving roles continuously juggle roles and responsibilities. Nurses working with women who are experiencing the debilitating effects of RA can be helpful in providing education or counseling that empowers women. Encouraging women to consider the importance of activities, the stress levels and the fulfillment they produce can assist them to negotiate or prioritize which roles to assume or avoid.

4. Support networks have been identified by other literature as a meaningful way to share illness experiences with those experiencing similar challenges. Using support groups as a form of education may be helpful to women who are trying to decide the value of taking-on and letting-go of roles that have been viewed as necessary.

5. The authors suggest caution in generalizing qualitative research findings. An important point they make is that what is identified in predominately Caucasian participants may be different from those of other ethnic or cultural backgrounds. Cultural competence is an important consideration for nurses as the usefulness of research findings are interpreted for various groups of women over time.

Activity 3

1. a. G
   b. B
   c. D
   d. A
   e. F
   f. D
   g. E
   h. G
   i. B

2. a. Credibility refers to qualitative research steps taken to ensure the accuracy, validity, and soundness of the data. Credibility can be confirmed when the research participants recognize the reported findings as their personal experience.

   b. Auditability is a research process that allows the work of a qualitative researcher or a person critiquing a research report to follow the thinking and/or conclusions of a researcher. The question of concern is whether the researcher(s) presented enough information for the reader to clearly understand the ways data were interpreted. When a data trail is auditable, it leads to the possibility of confirmability or an ability to clearly understand the ways the data were obtained, analyzed, and interpreted.

   c. Fittingness is the term used to answer these three questions: Are the findings applicable outside the study? Are the results or feelings meaningful to people not involved in the research? Are the findings meaningful to others who are in similar situations? Another idea closely related to fittingness is transferability; can the findings be translated into similar experiences in meaningful ways?

   d. Saturation refers to the point where data are being replicated in ways where no new ideas are coming forth about a specific concept or cultural phenomenon.

e. Trustworthiness implies that validity and reliability have been established and when a research report accurately represents or portrays the participants' experience.

Activity 4: Web-Based Activity

Your instructor may want to direct you to view some specific Internet links to learn additional specific aspects of qualitative research.

Activity 5: Evidence-Based Practice Activity

a. The quantitative aspect of this study examined relationships among social role quality, physical health, and psychological well-being in mid-life and late-life women diagnosed with RA.
b. The conclusion reached in the larger quantitative study was that women with RA who had positive social role experiences had less depression and more purpose in life despite physical difficulties than those who did not have positive role experiences.
c. Yes, the qualitative findings seemed to support what the quantitative findings suggested.
d. Unless you get the quantitative article and read it through, it will not be possible to truly understand what else might have been learned. One way of understanding the advantage to triangulated studies is by actually getting the reports from both aspects of the study and comparing what was learned. Although it might take a bit of effort to obtain this other study, it may be helpful in assisting you to better understand more about triangulated studies which can be important in building evidence-based knowledge for nursing practice.

CHAPTER 9

Activity 1

1. h
2. j
3. e
4. g
5. d
6. f
7. b
8. a
9. c

Activity 2

1. Testing. Taking the test repeatedly may be the factor leading to an increase in confidence and accuracy, rather than the experimental program. The use of different outcome instruments and measures may be necessary.
2. Instrumentation. The use of standardized calibrated equipment and training for the volunteers would increase the internal validity of the findings.

3. History. The increase in taxes could account for a decrease in the rate of cigarette smoking. Use of a control group and randomization would improve interpretation of the findings.

4. Selection bias. The differences in smoking cessation groups is needed to strengthen this design.

5. Mortality. The program is not successful for single homeless women with preschool children. It is important to look at the make-up of the final study sample when the results are interpreted.

6. Maturation. The mothers' confidence could be increased by any number of factors, including the act of caring for their infant during the months. The time of measurement could be immediately prior to discharge. Use of a control group would strengthen the findings.

Activity 3

a. The setting consisted of "...Community Health Services Division of the County Health Department in San Bernardino, California."

b. The subjects were144 pregnant adolescents.

c. The investigators outlined four criteria use to select the participants. The criteria for eligibility were 14-19 years of age; at 26 weeks gestation or less; having their first child; and planning to keep the infant. They excluded those adolescents who were dependent on narcotic or injection drugs, or were documented with a serious medical or obstetric problem.

d. No major area of information is missing. The investigators do note, however, that, "The complexities of obtaining medical records from multiple sources and providers made data collection of these data very difficult. As a result, a small portion of the infant health data were collected by maternal report only." Furthermore, they note that, "Evaluation of substance use was based on retrospective recall without the use of biochemical verification procedures." It would have increased the value of the study if periodic body fluid biochemical testing for drugs had been done.

e. Yes, the sample was homogenous for age and demographics in part due to clearly defined inclusion and exclusion criteria.

f. The variables were measured with a variety of measures including medical records, written questionnaires, observation scales, and structured interviews by nurses. Koniak-Griffin et al. thoroughly describe how they maintained constancy of data collection for both the EIP (experimental) and TPHNC (control group).

g. The TPHNC group who received traditional public health nursing care served as the control group.

Activity 4

1. Yes, the design is appropriate. The investigators were interested in evaluating the 2-year postbirth infant health and maternal outcomes of an early intervention program and used a randomized control trial to do this.

2. Yes, the methods used for control are consistent with the research design. Control is managed by ruling out extraneous or mediating variables that would compete with the independent variables as an explanation for a study's outcome. Koniak-Griffin et al. maintain

control of extraneous variables by using a homogenous sample, consistent data collection procedures, and manipulation of the independent variable and randomization of the sample into groups using a computer-based program.

3. This was an extremely complex and challenging study to conduct; it would require leadership by an experienced doctorally prepared researcher and a sophisticated and large research team. Examining the titles of the authors demonstrates the types of expertise and educational preparation needed by this team of researchers, which includes a doctorally prepared registered nurse who is the director of a research center, a postdoctoral fellow, a professor emeritus, a statistician, another doctorally prepared assistant professor, a doctoral student, and an administrative analyst. In addition, there would need to be a legion of data collectors, including public health nurses who had 60 hours training for the EIP intervention.

4. Yes, the parts of the study fit together and there is a logical flow to the design. The clinical concern and intervention is supported by the literature which links to the research objective and leads to the chosen design.

5. Threats to internal validity include history, maturation, instrumentation, mortality, and selection bias. The authors explained effectively how they controlled for maturation.

    History—The authors note no unanticipated events during the course of the study. This is difficult for the critiquer to evaluate because we are not given the dates when the study took place.

    Maturation—LoBiondo-Wood notes in Table 9-2 that in the Koniak-Griffin et al. study (2003) the lack of change in some of the variables and changes in other variables may have been due to the general maturation changes experienced by new mothers.

    Instrumentation—There is no reason to think that the instruments changed during the course of the study.

    Mortality—The investigators took the extra step of comparing sociodemographic characteristics (i.e., age, ethnicity/race, socioeconomic status, marital status, educational level, maternal acculturation, abuse history, length of gestation, and infant birth weight) between dropouts and study completers and found no significant differences.

    Selection bias—Koniak-Griffin et al. established criteria for selection of subjects and had an experimental and control group.

6. Threats to external validity include selection, reactive effects, and effects of testing.

    Selection—Koniak-Griffin et al. note that their sample was comprised predominantly of Latina adolescents, which limits generalization; however, it is important that this cultural group is being studied. The authors do not discuss the influence of culture on the intervention.

    Reactive effects—It is possible that there could have been some positive outcomes simply from being included in the study. Koniak-Griffin et al. note: "In an attempt to minimize participant attrition, the PHNs maintained regular telephone contact with adolescents in both groups throughout the 1st year postpartum. These interactions may have unintentionally served as an intervention."

Effects of testing—The instruments that were given at more than one point in the study were the HOME scale (used at 12 and 24 months) to measure the overall quality of the child's home environment, and the Nursing Assessment Teaching scale. The scales were administered by PHN evaluators rather than being completed by the subjects (adolescent mothers). This avoided the threat of subjects' responses being affected by taking a pretest.

The two additional measures—the CLSS and the SSI, which comprise external social competence and were administered at intake and 6 weeks postpartum—could have been at risk for measurement effects.

Activity 5: Web-Based Activity

It is possible to ascertain from the titles whether a study was most likely qualitative or quantitative. Based on the title alone, the study "Terminal illness experiences in older Japanese Americans" would most likely be qualitative. Another study, "How nursing affects the volume-outcomes relationship" presumably is a quantitative study because of the word "affects," which indicates measuring or testing of an outcome. However, some of the funded projects do not appear to be either quantitative or qualitative. The item "Advanced training in nursing outcomes research" could be a training grant to train nurses, or it could be a quantitative study measuring the outcomes of advanced training. However, this is an excellent site to learn about the most current funded research studies that are taking place. If you find a topic that is of interest to you, you may want to look for an article by the author, or if it is not yet published, you could contact the author as their university affiliation is listed.

Activity 6: Evidence-Based Practice Activity

1. C
2. C
3. C
4. C
5. B, C
7. A

CHAPTER 10

Activity 1

1. Experimental
2. Solomon four-group design
3. Time series design
4. After-only experiment
5. After-only nonequivalent control group design
6. True experiment
7. Nonequivalent control group design

Activity 2

1. Randomized control trial. After obtaining informed consent, subjects were randomly assigned to one of two groups using a computer-based program.
2. Experimental
3. a. Antecedent variables include ethnicity, age, educational value, and marital status. The authors note that they checked on these variables and found the group comparable on these variables which reduces the threat to internal validity.
   b. Intervening variables include change of health care status in any of the participants, the utilization of alcohol or drugs by the mother, or a change in the partner status of the mother.
4. The evidence provided by the findings of the study helps public health nurses make early intervention program versus traditional public health nursing care program resource allocation decisions with more certainty.

Activity 3

1.

	Pretest	Teaching	Post-Test
Group A	X	X	X
Group B		X	X
Group C	X		X
Group D			X

Note: The groups may be arranged in any order, but the four-group pattern must be followed.

2. The nurses would be randomly assigned to each of the groups using a table of random numbers or computer random assignment.
3. The pain knowledge and attitudes questionnaire would be used as a pretest.
4. The teaching program is the experimental treatment.
5. The pain knowledge and attitudes questionnaire is also the post-test or outcome measure.
6. The Solomon four-group design is ideal for experimental studies in which the pretest might affect the outcome. In this case, the questionnaire might change nurses' knowledge and attitudes about pain management. The researcher will be able to compare results for nurses receiving the teaching and not receiving the teaching with and without the pretest.
7. This type of design is particularly effective in ruling out threats to internal validity that the before-and-after groups may experience. It is effective for highly sensitive issues which might be affected by simply completing a questionnaire as a baseline pretest.
8. A disadvantage of the Solomon four-group design is that a large number of subjects must be available for assignment into the four groups.

Activity 4

1. a. Quasiexperimental, nonequivalent control group design.
   b. The presence of a pretest allows the investigator to compare the two groups on important antecedent variables before the intervention (treatment variable) is implemented.

c.   Minimal confidence that the intervention (treatment) group and the comparison con- trol) group were similar at the beginning of the study.

2.   a.   Quasiexperimental; interrupted time series design with a nonequivalent control group. If you indicated: (a) it was some type of a time series design, and (b) the com- parison group could not be considered equivalent to the treatment group because of the different data collection periods and methods, you have captured the essence of the design.

b.   To quote the investigators: "Anecdotal evidence of the positive effects of the TTM [the thermal mattress] on the body temperatures of VLBW [very-low-birth-weight] infants made it unethical to withhold its use; therefore, randomization was not pos- sible." (L'Herault, Petroff, Jeffrey, 2001, p. 212)

3.   a.   Time series design

b.   This type of design is useful in determining trends. Data are collected for a baseline, the experimental treatment is introduced and data are collected multiple times after- ward to determine a change from baseline. In longitudinal studies each subject can be compared with himself over time to allow trends to be observed. In this study, follow- up data were only collected twice. If there had been more data collection points, that would have helped to rule out alternative explanations for the results such as history effects.

c.   The disadvantages of this quasiexperimental design are that threats of selection and maturation cannot be ruled out, as well as there is a testing threat to validity due to multiple data collection points.

Activity 5

1.   Quasiexperimental designs are usually more practical, more feasible, and more adaptable to real-world practice. In many studies important to nursing, it is not possible to random- ize subjects into groups for practical or ethical reasons.

2.   The researcher must carefully examine other factors that could account for differences between groups.

3.   The clinician must carefully critique the research study and also look for other factors which might explain the results of the study. The results of any study with any design must be evaluated to determine if other factors influence the findings. The results should also be compared with the findings of other similar studies.

Activity 6: Web-Based Activity

1.   This number will vary depending on when the search is conducted.

2.   This is not an actual study but a review article. The authors state that "the purpose of the presentation is to identify various approaches to the design of control groups in experi- mental studies."

3.   This number will vary depending on when the search is conducted.

4.   This is a secondary analysis of a clinical trial which points out the importance of setting limits so that you narrow your search to the types of items that you desire.

Activity 7: Evidence-Based Practice Activity

1. Level 2
2. Level 3

CHAPTER 11

Activity 1

```
L O N G I T U D I N A L D M E
C I S P U E Q W H X O I Y H X
C R F L G Y Q E R C X E C G P
U W O L Z S B Q F H V O H H O
N T L S C I S Z A R R O I U S
L G T R S D L D U R Z L D O T
U E I O I S Q S E D L V W O F
I U W S J J E L O S Y U H I A
G T D K X O A C I E M D I I C
Q W R E E T O K T T E S T A T
A S A M I K E N B I B H U L O
D U O O K L H N P H O B Z V F
M C N G U L U E O L Y N R K C
K A M F G U P Q S B Z L A H T
L W J F V N E W J S W L E L V
```

1. Survey
2. Longitudinal
3. Correlational
4. Ex post facto
5. Cross-sectional
6. Correlational
7. Longitudinal
8. Survey
9. Cross-sectional
10. Cross-sectional

Activity 2

	Advantages	Disadvantages
Correlation studies	A3	D1, D3, D4, D7
Cross-sectional	A1, A8	D2, D5
Ex post facto	A4	D1, D2, D3, D4, D5, D7
Longitudinal	A2, A6	D2, D8, D9
Prospective	A2, A7	D3, D4, D7, D8
Retrospective	A4	D1, D2, D3, D4, D5, D7
Survey	A1	D5, D7

Activity 3
1. Longitudinal, Survey descriptive
2. Cross-sectional, Survey comparative
3. Longitudinal, Survey comparative. The term "longitudinal" most often is used when investigators collect data from a group three or more times. Data were collected in this study only twice, but there was a span of time between the two measures, and the investigators were describing change over time.
4. Survey descriptive or Survey exploratory
5. Survey descriptive
6. Methodological
7. Meta-analysis

Activity 4
1. Design descriptive, exploratory
2. Yes, one of the major points of the text authors was that consumers must be wary of non-experimental studies that make causal claims about the findings unless a causal modeling technique is used, which was not used in the Mohr study. It appears that the author may have attempted to state that a cause-and-effect relationship among the variables exists, which is not appropriate for an exploratory, nonexperimental study.

Activity 5
Ex post facto design

Activity 6: Web-Based Activity
1. Answers for this activity will vary depending on when the search is conducted.
2. Answers for this activity will vary depending on when the search is conducted.
3. Answers for this activity will vary depending on when the search is conducted.

Activity 7: Evidence-Based Practice Activity
1. d
2. b
3. a, b

CHAPTER 12

Activity 1
1. N
2. N
3. P
4. N
5. P
6. P
7. P

Activity 2
1. b
2. f
3. d
4. a
5. c
6. d
7. e
8. d

Activity 3
1. a. Yes, the sample is adequately described. The inclusion criteria were noted as patients who were aware of their diagnosis, had treatment and consultation, were able to read and speak English, showed no evidence of mental confusion, and were in a relationship.
    b. No, all men with prostate cancer were not included in the study, only those who met inclusion criteria.
    c. Convenience sampling
    d. Nonprobability
    e. Yes, the sample size could be considered adequate.
2. Uses most accessible persons/participants in this study and the ease of obtaining subjects.
3. Limits the generalizability of findings to others and applying findings to others. Further, the risks of bias are greater.
4. If a nurse is interested and has identified a problem in his or her practice, a convenience sample could be feasible for the initial study. This convenience sample supported the need for further study on the plan of care for patients with the diagnosis of prostate cancer. In terms of practice, it suggests that informational support given early in a diagnosis could support decision-making and lessen stress to the individual and significant other.

Activity 4
1. True
2. True
3. False

4. False
5. True
6. True
7. False

Activity 5

1. Yes, the characteristics of the sample were well-described.
2. Yes, the parameters of the population for this study would be children with the diagnosis of acute lymphocytic leukemia (between the age of 4 to 17 years of age)in three counties in California.
3. The sample is representative and encourages the reader to become familiar with the population and supportive of the needs of this identified group. The sample was from 95 English- and Spanish-speaking children in three southern California hospitals and their English- and Spanish-speaking parents. The authors note that the data reflected the demographics of the three counties in which the facilities are located.
4. The criteria were specific and inclusive of English- and Spanish-speaking children (between the ages of 4-17) and parents accessing care at the three centers of the study. The important issue was that they were recruited early in their diagnosis (within 1 month). Also, the exclusion criteria were specific.
5. Based on the material provided in the article, you could answer yes. The delimitation or exclusion criteria specified another chronic illness associated with pain, a fulminating disease, known cognitive disability, or inability to cope with the burden of research tasks as determined by the primary nurse.
6. Yes, it may be possible to replicate the study sample if there were similar populations available in the proposed study geographic areas.
7. The sample was obtained from the pediatric oncology populations of three facilities in southern California, using the Children's Oncology Group protocols. Yes, the method was appropriate for a longitudinal, descriptive design.
8. I cannot delineate any bias that appears evident. However, it is useful to consider that the instruments were in English and Spanish but no mention was made of the interviewers being able to speak Spanish. It is helpful to have interviewers or research associates who speak Spanish when dealing with families whose predominant language is Spanish. Most definitely, the introductions and interviews should have been done by a researcher or associate with the ability to speak Spanish for positive interaction and reliability. It would have been helpful for the authors to discuss the ability of interviewers to speak Spanish.
9. The sample size appears appropriate for a descriptive study and representative of the population in the three counties in southern California. The appropriateness of sampling strategy is validated by the analysis that found no differences between facility samples in terms of age, gender, or type of leukemia, thus allowing the authors to merge the data from the three sites for further analyses.
10. Yes, approval was obtained from the institutional review board of each facility. In accordance with consent, permission from parents and children for both instruments completion and interviews were obtained.

11. Yes they defined the limitations of this study. They mentioned that the findings could not be applicable to other types of childhood cancer. The investigators did confirm that the results were in accordance with other studies on cancer-related pain at diagnosis and during the course of treatment.

12. The authors mentioned at the end of the discussion section that because of the focus on leukemia, this precludes generalization of the findings to other types of childhood cancer. Although they do not propose replication with other samples, it can be inferred that to generalize the findings, this would be necessary.

Activity 6: Web-Based Activity

1. 59.5%
2. 32.4%
3. It appears to include data for all ages of people living in California.
4. In Table 1, chapter 12, it indicates in the Ethnicity Demographic Characteristic that the samples consisted of 31.6% Whites and 50.5% Hispanics. These demographics are different than the State of California demographics, which for the 2000 Census were 59.5% Whites and 32.4% Hispanic. However, it is important to note the study data was just for children between the ages of 4 to 17 years and the census data is for Californians of all ages. In order to correctly answer the question whether the samples data was representative of all Californians, then we would need to know the census data for California children between the ages of 4 and 17 years.

Activity 7: Evidence-Based Practice Activity

The sample and sampling strategy is one variable that will influence the strength of the evidence provided by the study. The evidence from a meta-analysis of all <u>randomized</u> controlled trials is more influential in making practice change decisions than from a single descriptive or qualitative study with a convenience sample.

CHAPTER 13

Activity 1

1. Nursing research committee
2. Institutional review board
3. Justice
4. Expedited review
5. Unethical research study
6. HIPAA

Activity 2

1. Beneficence
2. Justice
3. Respect for person

Activity 3

Elements of Informed Consent
1. √ Title of protocol
2. √ Invitation to participate
3. 0 Basis for subject selection
4. √ Overall purpose of the study
5. √ Explanation of benefits
6. √ Description of risks and discomforts
7. √ Potential benefits
8. 0 Alternatives to participation
9. √ Financial obligations
10. √ Assurance of confidentiality
11. 0 In case of injury compensation
12. 0 HIPAA disclosure
13. √ Subject withdrawal
14. √ Offer to answer questions
15. √ Concluding consent statement
16. √ Identification of investigators

Activity 4
1. The elderly
2. Children
3. Pregnant women
4. The unborn

Other correct responses include those who are emotionally or physically disabled, prisoners, the deceased, students, and people with AIDS.

Activity 5
1. a, c, d, f, g
2. a, b, c, d, f, g (Also, presume "e" was not adhered to because the study began in 1932 before IRBs and formal consent were required.)

Activity 6
1. Appendix A, Koniak-Griffin et al., in the "Procedure" section under "Methods," write, "After securing writing informed consent in accordance with the university Internal Review Board requirements for pregnant minors…" The authors demonstrate that they obtained informed consent and recognized the additional precautions needed because they were working with a vulnerable population.
2. Appendix B, Van Cleve et al. document in the "Data Collection Procedure," section of the article that institutional review board approval was obtained from each of the three facilities. In addition, they fully explain that permission for this vulnerable group (children) was obtained from parents and assent was obtained from the children. The authors have credibly explained their adherence to ethical research procedures.

3. Appendix C, Plach et al. report in the "Method" section that "Institutional Review Board approval was obtained for all study procedures."

4. Appendix D, Davison et al. note in the "Procedure" section of the article that "Data collection commenced following ethical approval of the study protocol by the appropriate institutional review committees. The first author provided an explanation of the purpose of the study and obtained written consent from each participant who had made an appointment at the Prostate Centre to access information."

Activity 7: Web-Based Activity

1. National Cancer Institute

2. Yes, because it is a government website supported by the U.S. National Institutes of Health.

Activity 8: Evidence-Based Practice Activity

You could check the Federal Register or other government documents or websites to determine if misconduct had occurred, or check the journal for a correction or follow-up research report.

CHAPTER 14

Activity 1

Study 1 (Koniak-Griffin et al.)

1. b, c, d, e

2. *Records of available data* were reviewed to determine visits to the ER and hospitalizations. Records were used as a way to verify information obtained from the mothers during the interviews.

Questionnaires were used to collect basic information about a variety of variables. Some of these variables could be difficult for individuals to discuss during an interview (e.g., sexual history). The questionnaire was a less intrusive instrument.

Observational—Trained observers viewed videotapes of interactions.

Interviews—The adolescent mothers were interviewed by PHNs who did not know whether the person interviewed was part of the control or intervention group.

Using a variety of methods allows researchers (and consumers) to have greater faith in the results when they are consistent across measures. The investigators specified why they chose some methods (e.g., the questionnaires), but did not offer the same explanation for each method. This is a very complex study with many methods; consequently, it is possible that the rationale for some methods were edited out to shorten the article.

Study 2 (Van Cleve et al.)

1. c

2. Children were interviewed using specific instruments to measure specific aspects of the pain experience. Parents responded for the younger children. The instruments were explained with information regarding previous use which served as the rationale for their use in this study.

3. It is believed to have been a successful data-collection method. The instruments were appropriate for the age groups. They were administered by individuals who were familiar with the instruments and were reviewed by others establishing interrater reliability.

Study 3 (Plach et al.)

1. c

2. The researchers wanted to "explore in greater depth the nature of social role experiences for women living with RA" (p. 34 in the original published article). They were exploring specific areas of information that had been the focus of the earlier quantitative study, so it made sense to structure the interviews to some degree while letting the subjects elaborate in other areas.

Study 4 (Davison et al.)

1. c, d

2. The men and their partners were included if they could read and write and assistance was available for the computerized portion of the data collection. Given the age of the participants, there may be some questions about any difficulties posed by the computerized parts of the interview. It is possible that the participants had had minimal experience with computers, but those conducting the interviews were there to provide assistance as needed.

Activity 2

1. Consumers
2. Physiological
3. Reactivity
4. Interviews
5. Records
6. Questionnaire
7. Objectivity, consistency
8. Concealment
9. Interrater reliability
10. Operationalization
11. Likert scale
12. Content analysis
13. Fun

```
D E L I V E R S T A T I S T C S Y E S P A S
S S A C A B I N E T F O R K A Z O S P E I O
I A W O P E R A T I O N A L I Z A T I O N B
G T S N O R N E V E R B Y D N E A U X B T J
N S Y S T E M A T I C A J H T B S D V S E E
I F L I K E R T S C A L E E R R O Y A E R C
F A K S C A L E S N O V N O C A A U L R R T
H C U T A C R A T I M A P V E T P U I V A I
Y T B E B H I R T E M A H V W K I C D A T V
P C O N T E N T A N A L Y S I S P V O T E I
R O Y C B K D S I S R T S A D V A N E I R T
E R E Y O D U G K A T P I B I O I O G O R Y
A V S I B R Q U E S T I O N N A I R E N E C
C I A R E S E A R C H L R E A C E S O L O
T O B M E X C E L A E O O D A T A C O V I N
I U E A E V A L I D S T G N O S T O O E A S
V N Y E S S I N T E R V I E W S A R F R B U
I H A P P I E N E S S P C A T A G D U N I M
T X C I T E D E L P H I A T O T P S N V L E
Y C E A T U B B S A N D L D O N N M A R I R
Y A B L E A C O N C E A L M E N T O O T T S
A I K E V A L I K E I I A B C O N S U M Y S
```

Activity 3

1. Children; interactions between people where the investigator is not part of the interaction; psychiatric patients; classrooms
2. The consent is usually of the type where permission to observe for a specified purpose is requested. The specific behaviors that are to be observed are not named. The use of the data and degree of anonymity are explained. In some situations, the subjects will be asked to review the data after the observation and before inclusion in the data pool.
3. Reactivity is the major concern, when the investigator has reason to believe that his or her presence will change the nature of the subjects' behavior.

Activity 4

Physiological measures would be of minimal use since the data being sought would not involve actual measures of the residents' physiological status. Not particularly interested in current blood pressure, temperature, urinary output, etc.

Could consider using observation; e.g., sitting in an emergency room and observing the types of health care concerns that enter. Would need to think about whether this would be observation with concealment. Would need to wrestle with the notion of what is private information and what is public domain information.

Could use questionnaires and collect data from all types of health care providers. Could provide a lot of data in a short time. Wonder how busy they would be and what would be the probability of their filling out the questionnaire?

Could use an interview. Is costly in terms of researcher time, but could provide more detailed information because subjects could be asked to expand upon specific items. But who should be interviewed? How does one get into their offices/homes, etc.?

Need to get some information from the people who actually live here. Wonder how a cross-section of those individuals could be reached? Could they be called? What about those people without a telephone?

Better check out the census data to get a clearer picture of what is being dealt with. Probably have some morbidity and mortality data collected by the state health department. Would probably utilize existing records to get a first sense of what the parameters of "health" are in this community. Then talk to some people about who knew the most about this area and arrange some interviews with these individuals. These would be guided interviews with open-ended items to encourage the sharing of as much information as possible. Would also seek a way to collect data from a variety of health care users; e.g., surveys in the waiting room of various agencies, maybe the crowd at a mall, at a county fair.

One data collection instrument would not be sufficient to collect the information needed about the areas addressed.

Activity 5

1. d
2. a
3. d
4. a, b, c
5. d

Activity 6: Web-Based Activity

1. NDNQI—National Database of Nursing Quality Indicators
2. Ten quality indicators form the core.
3. Form would be categorized as a survey.

Activity 7: Evidence-Based Practice Activity

1. The methodology used in the *JAMA* study was "subjective daily symptom scores" for nine cold symptoms. No difference was found in the duration of symptoms between those who used the zinc lozenges and those who did not.
2. It is doubtful that one would change a practice to the point of insisting that everyone with a cold should be encouraged to use zinc lozenges, but it is also doubtful that one would ask patients NOT to use the lozenges. It is one study, and one would want to look for more evidence before either encouraging or discouraging the use of these lozenges.

CHAPTER 15

Activity 1

1. S; avoided by proper calibration of the scale.

2. S; decrease error by providing instructions, ensuring confidentiality, or other means to allow students to freely express themselves.
3. R; lessen by training research assistants and using strict protocols or rule books to guide analysis.
4. R; decrease their anxiety by addressing their concerns, providing comfort measures, or other efforts that might decrease their anxiety. Anxiety may alter the test responses.

Activity 2
1. Construct validity; construct validity
2. Face validity
3. Content validity
4. Context experts
5. Construct validity or convergent validity
6. Convergent validity; contrasted groups; divergent validity; factor analysis; hypothesis testing
7. Content validity

Activity 3
1. Stability; homogeneity; equivalence
2. Test-retest methods could be accomplished by giving the same test again at a later date and seeing if the two scores are highly correlated. Parallel or alternate forms, such as alternate versions of the same test, could also be used to establish stability.
3. Alternate forms would be better if the test-taker is likely to remember and be influenced by the items or the answers from the first test.
4. a. 2
   b. 4
   c. 1
   d. 3
5. a. Yes, these instruments had face validity. The researchers were addressing stress and coping following a prostate cancer diagnosis. How patients and partners prefer to make decisions, how to manage information, specific information needs, how individuals were feeling, and depressive feelings in cancer patients were the topics of interest, and the instruments appeared to be appropriate to address these issues.
   b. Was developed to measure depressive symptoms in general population. Had been adapted for use with cancer patients. Specific information about the scoring was provided. A measure of reliability was provided.
   c. The information provided for all instruments would increase confidence in the results of the study. They were appropriate. Measures were taken to provide assistance with a minimum of interference with information obtained. If I were interested in this clinical area and had skimmed this study, this would be one that I would go back and read in more detail.

Activity 4
Current smoker, B/P screening, height, weight, BMI, and several demographic variables

Activity 5

Critiquing Questions

Instrument	#1	#2	#3	#4	#5	#6	#7	#8
Poker Chip	N	?	Y	?	?	N	N	?
Preschool Body Outline	N	?	?	?	?	N	N	?
Adolescent Pediatric Pain	Y	Y	Y	Y	?	N	N	?
Dot Matrix	N	N	Y	?	?	N	N	?
Pediatric Pain Coping	Y	Y	N	N	?	N	N	?
Perception of Management Effectiveness	N	N	N	N	?	N	N	N
Functional Status	Y	Y	Y	?	?	N	N	?

Activity 6: Evidence-Based Practice Activity

First, this study would need to be put into context. It would need to be known what other studies were available in the same area. If a decision were being made based solely on the published reliability and validity information, it would not be considered a strong study.

To qualify this statement, there may be more information about the reliability and validity of the instruments. Some of it may have been cut to meet required article length. Some information is given, and what is presented is valuable and does lead to some confidence in the results—certainly more confidence than if they had been using several newly constructed instruments.

A final answer would be "it depends." Some questions would need to be asked and more listening would need to be done.

CHAPTER 16

Activity 1

You will have your set of completed cards.

Activity 2

1. d
2. c
3. d
4. a
5. a, b, or c, depending on the tool used to measure satisfaction
6. a

7. b
8. d
9. a
10. c

Activity 3

Across
1. j   Goofy's best friend
3. e   Old abbreviation for mean
5. b   Abbreviation for number of measures in a given data set (the measures may be individual people or some smaller piece of data like blood pressure readings)
8. m   Describes a set of data with a standard deviation of 3 when compared with a set of data with a standard deviation of 12
10. h   Abbreviation for standard deviation
11. f   Marks the "score" where 50% of the scores are higher and 50% are lower
12. c   Measure of variation that shows the lowest and highest number in a data set

Down
1. l   The values that occur most frequently in a data set
2. i   68% of the values in a normal distribution fall between ±1 of this statistic
4. d   Can describe the height of a distribution
6. g   Describes a distribution characterized by a tail
7. k   Very unstable
9. a   Measure of central tendency used with interval of ratio data

Activity 4
1. a. overweight or obesity
   b. nominal
2. a. educational intervention
   b. weight gain
   c. intervention = nominal
      weight = ratio
3. a. IVs = postpartum stress scores
   b. depression scores

Activity 5
1. Null hypothesis
2. ANOVA; parametric statistics
3. Research hypothesis
4. Sampling error
5. Parameter; sample
6. Correlation
7. Type II error; Type I error

8. Probability
9. Practical significance
10. Nonparametric statistics
11. Statistical significance
12. Research hypothesis; null hypothesis
13. c, b, a, e, d

Activity 6

1. Whether the childbirth experience or the preferred gender of the baby had an effect on the postpartum health scores
2. n or the number of subjects in each category and the means and standard deviations of the scores on the postpartum health scale
3. *t* test
4. IV = childbirth experience, gender preferences; DV = postpartum health score
5. IV = nominal; DV = interval
6. There was no difference in postpartum health scores based on childbirth experience. There was no difference in postpartum health scores based on gender preference.

Activity 7

1. a. yes
   b. yes
   c. yes
   d. yes
2. All four studies used descriptive statistics to describe certain characteristics of the sample (e.g., age, sex, ethnicity).
3. Yes for all four studies.
4. The Van Cleve et al. study—because the purpose of the study was to describe the pain experiences of the children using a specific model.
5. a. yes
   b. yes
   c. no
   d. yes
6. a. Chi square was used to compare the EIP group to the traditional PHN care group on the variables of: (a) immunization rates for infants, (b) maternal substance abuse, (c) educational outcomes, and (d) repeat pregnancies. ANOVA was used to analyze internal social competence, external social competence, NCATS scores, and HOME scores between the two groups.
   b. *t* test was used to analyze the difference in coping strategies used when grouped by age, gender, number of strategies used. *t* test also used to compare pain intensity scores before and after management when grouped by age and specific interview. *t* test used to compare functional status at different interview times. *r* was used to explore the relationship between the pain intensity scores after management and the management effectiveness scores. Mann-Whitney *U* was used to compare perception of management effectiveness between Latino and White children.

c. Not applicable, since this is a qualitative study
d. Chi square was used to analyze the PLAN for active role in decision-making with the ACTUAL role in decision-making in consideration of the variables of age, education, status of treatment, and decision-making. Also used in the analysis of:
   - Roles patient preferred for partner and roles patients thought partners actually played
   - Treatment status and education and roles for partners
   - Preferences of partners for own role in decision-making

ANOVA was used when the analysis looked at the interplay of levels of anxiety, depression, and the role assumed in decision-making. Paired *t* test was used to analyze the differences between the pre- and post-test scores of state anxiety and depression.

7. The answers to this question may vary.

Activity 8: Web-Based Activity

1. Data about a blue whale: heart weighs 0.5 ton and the circulatory system contains 2,000 gallons of blood.
2. 44% of women who are murdered by their intimate partner had visited an ED within the past 2 years, and 93% had had at least one injury visit to an ED at some time.

Activity 9: Evidence-Based Practice Activity

ED nurses should stop and consider how their actions in the ED could make a difference. They could check out the websites that are listed as references on the CDC site and look for recommendations of experts in the field. They could anticipate finding guidelines for ways of interviewing injured women that would increase the probability of uncovering IPV. They could make sure that literature about IVP and safe places were readily available in the ED. They may also need to devise a way to keep some data so there could be some evaluation of the steps they had taken (such as by asking someone in the local school of nursing to work with them on this task).

CHAPTER 17

Activity 1

1. R
2. D
3. R
4. D
5. R
6. R
7. R
8. D
9. D
10. D

Activity 2
1. Yes.
    - The table supplements and economizes the text. It would probably require about two pages of text to put all of the information in narrative form.
    - The title and headings are clear.
    - Does not repeat the information included in the text.
2. Cereal was eaten most often.
3. Girls drank more orange juice.
4. 10th graders declined to answer the questions most often.

Activity 3
Answers will vary from class to class.

Activity 4
1. a. Number of men = 74 and the number of partners = 74
    b. Partners
    c. Standard deviation (SD) of 6.9 and 8.8
2. a. All values decreased
    b. No (look at the last sentence of the paragraph below the table)
3. 101
4. 3

Activity 5: Web-Based Activity
1. The rating should be a 1; there were too many items to even think about reviewing, and there was very little consistency in the content among the items.
2. This answer will vary depending on when the search was conducted.

Activity 6: Evidence-Based Practice Activity
Answers will vary depending on when the website was accessed, and personal experience.

CHAPTER 18

Please note that what follows are the results of one inspectional reading of the Koniak-Griffin et al. article. You are not expected to agree with these findings. Some of you may agree, but many of you will not.

Systematic skimming: In reading the title, the fairly long abstract, the biographies, and the discussion, the following conclusions were made:
1. Yes, I am interested in adolescents, so this population is one that would attract me.
2. The clinical area is tangentially related to an interest of mine.
3. I would proceed to superficial reading.

Superficial reading:

1. Remembered about the study:
   - Home visitation was the treatment.
   - Public health nurses were trained.
   - These data were based in a longitudinal study.
   - Social competence was the driving theory.
   - There is some concern about contamination between the two groups of mothers. Not sure about some treatment effects.
   - Instruments OK—used in other studies.
   - Data appeared to be OK.
   - The results were OK.
2. Conclusion: I would reread this study in greater detail. It contains some nuggets that could support some interests of mine. It would not be directly related to my research interests, but is interesting enough to be useful.

Remember the purpose of inspectional reading is to decide what to do about further reading of the study. What did you decide?

CHAPTER 19

Activity 1
1. B
2. A
3. C
4. B
5. D
6. D
7. A

Activity 2
1. Conceptual
2. policies; procedures
3. a. rationale linear approach
   b. transitional tradition
   c. transformational change
4. problem-focused
5. stakeholder
6. patient or population, intervention, comparison, outcome
7. a. methods for noting the type of research
   b. how to rate the quality of individual articles
   c. grading the strength of the body of evidence
8. synthesis

Activity 3

a. 1
b. 4
c. 6
d. 11
e. 12
f. 2
g. 5
h. 8
i. 10
j. 3
k. 7
l. 9

Activity 4

1. Include the EBP terminology into the mission, vision, philosophy statements
2. Establish explicit performance expectations about EBP for staff at all levels
3. Integrate the work of EBP into the governance structure of nursing departments and the health care system
4. Recognize and reward EBP behaviors
5. a. Volunteer to serve on a committee that is reviewing the mission, vision, etc. of the agency or the unit
    b. Ask to read the mission, vision, and philosophy and ask about EBP
6. a. Volunteer to help evaluated evidence-based changes in practice
    b. Ask questions!
    c. Think about how to improve practice
    d. Reward nurses who ask practice questions
7. a. Look for ways to work with other disciplines to implement EBP
    b. Volunteer to be a "guinea pig" for an interdisciplinary project
    c. Volunteer to serve on the committee to select/change documentation of care systems
8. a. Create a "These People Did Something Great" bulletin board
    b. Consider adding EBP activities to the career ladder/merit considerations

Activity 5

1. There are three recommendations:
    - The use of nurse-led clinics is recommended for patients with coronary heart disease (Grade B).
    - The use of nurse-led clinics may increase clinic attendance and follow-up rates (Grade B).
    - Nurse-led clinics are recommended for patients who require lifestyle changes to decrease their risk of adverse outcomes associated with coronary heart disease (Grade A).

2. The article was published in South Australia.
3. The article's original probably would not influence the use of the review.

CHAPTER 20

Activity 1

Item #	Patient "P"	Intervention "I"	Compare "C"	Outcome "O"
#1	Parents	Recliners	Convert-O-Beds	More parents stay
#2	Hemodialysis clients	Verbal instruction + take-home materials	Verbal instruction only	Decrease in adherence difficulties
#3	Children	No vending machines	Vending machines	Decrease in weight of children

Activity 2
Answers will vary.

Activity 3
Tool #1: PICO
Tool #2: librarian, information literacy
Tool #3: screening questions
Tool #4: therapy studies; meta-analysis; harm articles; confidence interval; relative risk reduction; likelihood ratios
Tool #5: none

Activity 4
1. Therapy
2. Diagnosis
3. Prognosis
4. Harm
5. Therapy
6. Therapy
7. Therapy
8. Therapy
9. Prognosis
10. Prognosis (could also be classified as Harm)
11. Diagnosis
12. Harm

Activity 5: Web-Based Activity

1. $25.00 per systematic review ($265 for an individual subscription)
2. A long list of titles of reviews appears first; an abstract of the systematic review appears next
3. Bottom line: is there is not enough information in this "little gem" for a practitioner to change his or her practice based on it alone.
4. Answers will vary.

NOTES

NOTES

NOTES

NOTES

NOTES

NOTES

NOTES